Elizabeth Ettorre has a P...
London School of Economics. She worked for 16 years as a
Research Sociologist at the University of London where she
carried out research into women, alcohol, illegal drugs and
HIV/AIDS. In 1991 she moved to Helsinki. In Finland, she
has been a Visiting Scholar in the Department of Sociology,
Åbo Akademi University; a guest lecturer in Sociology and
Women's Studies at a number of universities throughout the
country; and a Docent in Sociology at both Åbo Akademi
University and the University of Helsinki. Currently, she is
the Project Co-ordinator of a European Commission
research project, 'The development of pre-natal screening in
Europe: the past, the present and the future'.

Her other books include *Lesbians, Women and Society*
(1980), *Women and Substance Use* (1992) and *Gendered
Moods: Psychotropics and Society* (with Elianne Riska, 1995).

WOMEN &
ALCOHOL

A private pleasure or a public problem?

ELIZABETH ETTORRE

First published by The Women's Press Ltd, 1997
A member of the Namara Group
34 Great Sutton Street, London EC1V ODX

British Library Cataloguing-in-Publication Data
A catalogue record for this book is available from the British Library

ISBN 0 7043 4437 8

Typeset by FSH Print & Production
Printed and bound in Great Britain by Caledonian International

To my Beloved, with deep appreciation for giving her constant support as well as sharing her brilliant ideas and critical vision

ACKNOWLEDGEMENTS

During my 30-year career as a woman sociologist I have worked as an 'alcohol and drugs' researcher in three different societies: American, British and Finnish. Through my work, I have been lucky enough to observe the emergence of the American hippie, drug culture alongside its established temperance culture; the liberal, pop culture of the British; and the somewhat prescriptive, beer-drinking culture of the Finns. In all three countries, I have met and talked with countless numbers of women who have experienced both the pleasure and the pain of alcohol and drug use, and the physical, psychological, emotional and social harm it can cause. This book, focusing specifically on women and their use of alcohol, is a result of my personal work history which has been both deep and enriching, and is informed by my cross-cultural research experience.

There are many people who have given me support in writing this book. First, I would like to thank my editor at The Women's Press, Kathy Gale, who has provided not only constant support and encouragement during the writing of this book but also very insightful, editorial comments on the manuscript. Also, I would like to thank Hannah Kanter, who was my previous editor at The Women's Press and who contracted me to write this work.

I am also grateful to all the women who agreed to be interviewed and hope they find this book helpful to them in their own lives.

Since I have been in Finland, Elianne Riska from the Department of Sociology, Åbo Akademi University, has provided me with much valued, collegial support, and this ongoing collaboration is much appreciated. This book has also been influenced over the years by my fruitful discussions with men and women colleagues who have helped me to explore key theoretical and practical issues concerning women's use of alcohol and/or women's health. These colleagues include: Geoff Hunt, Susanne MacGregor, Shirley Otto, Hilary Rose, Meg Stacey, Mary Stewart, Mary Treacy and Jan Waterson. I should like to thank them for their encouragement and support of my work.

Of course, I am also most grateful to my nearest and dearest friends for their support and encouragement.

Elizabeth Ettorre
Helsinki, Finland

CONTENTS

CHAPTER 2   Multiple problems and women's drinking

CHAPTER 3   Multiple images and social hypocrisy

CHAPTER 4   Female 'treatment' or women-healing?

CHAPTER 5   Becoming strong: women-sensitivity and self-help

CHAPTER 6 Mixing women-sensitivity with alcohol: a Molotov cocktail?

INTRODUCTION

In writing this book, I want to address the issues related to how women use and abuse alcohol – a legal and socially accepted substance in many societies. The use of all kinds of substances, whether those which are medically addictive and lead to dependence and misuse such as alcohol, tranquillisers, heroin, and so on, or those which are psychologically addictive such as food, is important in the lives of most if not all women in our society.[1]

Breaking from traditions used by many of my colleagues working in this area, I would like this to be a book that combines women-sensitive ideas about women and alcohol with a broad, 'user friendly' approach. I want it to be of practical benefit to women who see themselves as having a problem with alcohol use. I would also like these ideas to help women, whether or not they experience difficulties with alcohol, to see the reasons why their use of alcohol is different from men's. Along with Sarah Hafner, I believe that the problems associated with alcohol 'flare up in men and women differently'.[2]

If we look at the issue of women and alcohol through the eyes of traditional sociology or alcohol research, we see that it is quite common for an author or a researcher to discuss this social issue solely from an academic viewpoint. There is little if any reference to how one feels. This is because academic viewpoints are supposed to be based on what is scientific. Scientific techniques have been developed to gather research and statistics, to create an awareness of the social issues authors or researchers examine, and to produce scientific facts. More often than not these facts are divorced from emotions, feelings and, as a result, people's lives. In my view, any work, scientific or otherwise, which excludes human feelings cannot allow for the growth of compassion: a sympathetic consciousness of others' suffering along with a desire to reduce it. The women and alcohol issue needs such a compassionate response.

Of course, it is interesting and worthwhile to develop a scientific viewpoint on the women and alcohol issue.[3] But this should not exclude other approaches that aim to create an understanding of the reality of our everyday lives as women who use alcohol.

It is a tragedy that alcohol is abused by some women. For me, however, it is a greater tragedy that while alcohol has had deep and sometimes symbolic meanings for women who experience problems with alcohol, these meanings are seldom understood in society.[4] As we shall see, women who abuse alcohol are seen as less than women. Society views them as 'alcoholics'[5] and therefore as abnormal, deviant, sick, selfish, evil and even promiscuous women. But the reasons why women may be 'alcoholics' or are over-drinking and misusing alcohol are often left out of society's picture.

WOMEN'S ALCOHOL USE IN PERSPECTIVE

If we look specifically at the women and alcohol issue, there are four problems, in my view, which need to be overcome before we are able to produce a women-sensitive approach. This approach aids an understanding of the fact that women are not only hurt by alcohol itself, but also by the lack of understanding of the issues related to their drinking.

First, traditional ideas on women and alcohol tend to present women as a uniform group. Differences amongst women remain hidden if not denied. In this type of homogeneous viewpoint, key social factors such as age, ethnic origins, able-bodiness, social class, race, sexual orientation and so on tend to be lost. If women are viewed as a homogeneous group, the problems women experience with alcohol cannot be treated effectively. For example, in social situations, the lesbian may experience her use of alcohol differently from a heterosexual, disabled woman. For many lesbians, drinking has become an acceptable social lubricant,[6] and drinking to the point of intoxication can be sometimes seen as acceptable at certain social events. On the other hand, a woman in a wheelchair may find that she needs to be in a social space where she can easily manoeuvre herself around a group of socialising people, so rather than intoxication, moderation is likely to be her rule. This sense of difference should be recognised and appreciated if women's problems with alcohol are to become more visible.

Second, research on women and alcohol has more often than not focused on treatment. Women already being treated or those seeking 'official' help tend to be looked upon as the representatives of women who experience negative drinking or problems with alcohol. This focus distorts our views on the women and alcohol issue. There are a number of women, possibly a larger number than we think, who experience negative drinking but who do not seek treatment. These women may be involved in self-help groups or Alcoholics Anonymous (AA). They may not be involved in any groups at all.

That official treatment may be refused or not even considered as a viable option for some women is an interesting issue that needs to be explored.[7] Is it because women fear the stigma of being labelled publicly an 'alcoholic' if they go into treatment? Is this risk too great for some women who are mothers? At the very least, while being outside of treatment and inside AA or contained within a self-help group, some women find anonymity. Are women afraid of losing their children, their jobs, their partners, their husbands, and so on, if they seek treatment? Do they have other types of support, such as friends, relatives, therapeutic networks or groups which they feel are more helpful to them than the official treatment system? These are questions that have not yet been answered in the area of women and alcohol and that I attempt to answer later in this book.

Third, if we do take a good look into official treatment systems, we see little attempt to develop or indeed to offer what I call an integrated approach, sensitive to women's needs and problems. Self-help groups or women-only groups can be a forceful means of support and change for women. There are a few enlightened services, for example in the USA, Britain and Australia, which attempt to meet women's needs in this way. Nevertheless, women's services tend to be seen as 'special services'. If there are financial cutbacks, these services are the first to be abolished. Catering to women's needs should be seen as essential in any treatment or rehabilitation service,[8] for example through the provision of women's groups and childcare. Unfortunately, this view is not held within the majority of treatment settings. It is therefore hardly surprising that many women do not seek official treatment and find help in other ways.

Fourth, we need to consider ways of making women's use of alcohol visible in social areas that have not been previously examined. Although it is interesting to know the numbers of women who have a drinking problem, the kinds of alcohol that women drink, the social characteristics of women who go into treatment, and so on, it can be very revealing to link women's use of alcohol to their experience of themselves as women in society. Concern about women's use of alcohol needs to address broad social issues and, furthermore, to make links between these broader issues and the roots of women's drinking. For example, can issues around how women experience their roles as women or the subtleties of power experienced in gender relations have an effect upon how they drink? Simply, we need to develop a more social view of the women and alcohol issue as a way of balancing the individualistic view offered traditionally by treaters and researchers. Only then will we come nearer to a true picture of women's use of alcohol.

WOMEN'S POSITIVE AND NEGATIVE DRINKING

Women drink alcohol in a variety of ways, for a variety of reasons and in a variety of situations. In this book, I put forward the view that among women who drink alcohol there is a difference between 'positive drinking'[9] and 'negative drinking'.

In using the terms 'negative' and 'positive' drinking, I am not imposing moral standards on women's drinking. I am not saying that those involved in positive drinking are better than those involved in negative drinking or that women who experience negative drinking should feel bad, guilty or negative about themselves as women. I have consciously avoided using the terms 'negative drinkers' and 'positive drinkers' as a way of imposing moral judgements on specific groups of women drinkers. Rather, I have focused on women's use of alcohol as being experienced either negatively or positively. Most important, I have developed this focus from the viewpoint of women who have these experiences, whether they encounter negative drinking or positive drinking. Here, the main point is that when women experience problems with their use of alcohol, this inevitably leads to disapproval, negative feelings and discontent within themselves. They may also find themselves judged harshly by others. Here, disapproval becomes the key issue. This is because all women, drinkers or non-drinkers, are constrained in many ways to conform to powerful social images, telling us what it means to be an 'acceptable woman' in society. Some, if not many, women fail in their attempts to reflect satisfactory female images or to embody femininity. This places a double burden on women who experience problems with alcohol. Not only do they suffer from disapproval and scorn, but also they appear to have failed as women.

Positive drinking

Positive drinking is primarily about moderate drinking; it describes when a woman drinks alcohol moderately during social and/or private occasions. She does not need to drink in excess to feel good. Alcohol is viewed as a relaxing substance and, most important, a woman knows when she has had enough alcohol to make her feel good. Her drinking alcohol becomes more of a positive than a negative experience. Along with moderation and feeling good, positive drinking may also involve actually enjoying the taste of alcohol. For example, one woman[10] reflecting on her use of alcohol says:

> I like now and then to have an alcoholic drink. I like to drink wine. I also like beer. I think I like it because I like the taste. But if I never had another drink in my life, it would not bother me. I do not really need it.

For others, moderate drinking is used as a social tool – to socialise. One woman described her positive drinking in this way:

> Alcohol has played a role in my life in social situations. I am a social drinker . . . when we have a special dinner or during the holidays we'll have a bottle of wine or maybe a couple of beers.

Now I would like to look more closely at women who experience positive drinking. Here I give some examples of positive drinking and then contrast them with examples of negative drinking.

A single, working-class mother works all week to support her three young children. On Saturday evenings, she goes to a pub or a bar with women friends to have a few beers. She finds the experience 'good', beneficial or enjoyable for her because it gives her a chance to see close friends she otherwise would not meet. The alcohol helps to liven things up and keep the conversation flowing. A single business-woman, a woman of colour, after coming home from a tiring workday, occasionally has a glass of wine with her evening meal. She enjoys the taste of good wine and is invited every year to attend a wine-tasting event at her local business association. A young, unemployed woman spends weekends at her male friend's apartment. Every Friday evening, they watch television together and drink a few glasses of rum and coke. A middle-aged housewife drinks a few cocktails, beer or wine with her husband during the week. She enjoys these moments because she is able to relax and be most herself. A lesbian goes every Sunday with her partner to have a special lunch with her mother. They drink wine and enjoy each other's company for a few hours.

All of the women described above are examples of women who experience positive drinking. Alcohol enhances their lives as women; they are able to drink alcohol in a controlled way, whether they are conscious of this or not. If alcohol were taken out of their lives, they would not experience too much suffering. Additionally, these women do not experience problems related to their use of alcohol. For them, alcohol as a social drug is a pleasurable experience.

If used in a controlled way, alcohol can have a useful role both socially and individually. Alcohol can be important as a social lubricant. It can help one to relax with others in a non-threatening manner. It allows one to create social spaces for communicating.

But it can also be described as a drug about which one needs to develop boundaries. One physical effect of alcohol for some women is that it makes them feel uninhibited. For example, alcohol helps some women to speak more freely, without fear, than if they were sober. This may make alcohol so attractive to them that it becomes difficult for them to develop what one woman described as 'one's own borders about alcohol' and other positive drinking skills such as when to drink, why, what is too much, and so on. One woman I spoke to believed that women should learn the difference between pleasure and need in their use of alcohol. She reflected on her youth when she learned how to drink positively for herself. In her view, this was a learning process, and developing the borders around alcohol was different for each woman. She says:

> I know when I first started going out, the greatest pleasure in my youth was to go to the pub, to order drinks and to drink them in the pub. When one gets to a certain age, drinking is like a ritual one goes through. The first thing one does is go out and have a good old drink with friends . . . Where is the border between drinking for pleasure – because you like the taste or you like the slight sensation of a few drinks, and drinking out of compulsion – because you need

it? Well, I think everyone has their own border. I have always been rather fortunate because too much alcohol does not agree with me. Usually, I feel sick before I get drunk. So then I stop drinking and say I have had enough.

Another woman described how she developed her own way of drinking through trial and error. Learning positive drinking was all about learning at what point she had had enough alcohol to feel pleasure. She believed that before learning about pleasure, a novice drinker had to test herself and learn the 'point to be reached' or where the border in fact was:

> When you first go out and order drinks, the barman gives them to you. You don't say no because you are under age or because you are not legally entitled to have a drink. Well I didn't. At that age, I'd never tried alcohol. So obviously you drink too much as most people do at that age. Then you wake up in the morning with a hangover and think, 'Oh my god! Is that it?' For me, I was learning about a point to be reached. Gradually you learn to know, 'My point is reached and I have had enough.' You have found your own border.

The message here is that all drinkers need to learn their own points to be reached – to develop their own borders in order to feel good – and to learn that pleasure should be a key to positive drinking. For some women, learning their own borders might mean that they will not drink alcohol because they cannot control their intake. Other women who like the effects of alcohol and who find pleasure in drinking and socialising with others may want to drink moderately. Drinking is a positive experience for them. However, one must not lose sight of the fact that some people are harmed by overdrinking, and it is this aspect of women's relationship to alcohol that the following discussion will address.

Negative drinking

A woman involved in negative drinking may experience multiple problems with her use of alcohol. She is likely to be unable to control her drinking, and this loss of control inevitably causes difficulties in her life. She needs to drink in excess to feel the effects of alcohol, but in the end these effects make her feel bad physically, psychologically, or emotionally.

One woman, who for many years found alcohol to be a problem in her life, spoke about her feelings. Her negative drinking was all about 'killing' bad feelings in her life and 'running' from pain. She saw this as a pattern for women who experience problems with their drinking:

> You find that there are lots of women who will drink heavily to avoid the pain of abuse in their lives – then there is something underneath it all . . . it means that if a woman is using the drug to kill the pain . . . she is not ready to face whatever the pain is . . .

This woman does not drink any longer 'to kill' her pain. In fact, she does not drink at all. She believes that women who drink too much usually do so because they cannot cope with their feelings, whatever these may be. In her eyes, alcohol was a negative part of her life. Unlike women who experience positive drinking and feel good, she needed to drink in excess to kill feelings. She felt bad if she allowed herself to feel at all. In the end, she used alcohol in the same way some use tranquillisers – to 'medicate' feelings.

Using similar social situations to those described above to illustrate positive drinking, let us now look at examples of women who experience negative drinking.

A single, working-class mother works all week to support her three young children. She is unable to cope with the stress both of working and taking care of her children. Every evening she buys at least four bottles of strong beer which she drinks after she has put her children to bed. When in her bed, she cries herself to a state of tiredness and keeps telling herself that beer helps her to sleep. A single businesswoman, a woman of colour, finds it difficult to cope with hidden racism she experiences at her workplace. Every day, when she comes home from work, she has a bottle of wine with her evening meal. She often goes to her local business club at the weekends to drink cocktails with her colleagues, but she returns home intoxicated. A young, unemployed woman finds it difficult to cope with her situation and uses most of her money to buy bottles of rum which she drinks alone in the evening. When she is drinking on weekends at her male friend's apartment, he often complains that she drinks too much. A middle-aged housewife hides a few bottles of Scotch in her house every week. Neither her husband nor her children know that she is drinking during the day. She feels ashamed. A lesbian has just publicly declared her sexuality at her university. She drinks every day before going to classes to cope with her anxiety. On Sunday, after having lunch with her mother, her partner has to drive them home, as she herself is over the acceptable alcohol limit to drive.

For the above women, their use of alcohol causes difficulties in their lives. While their social situations are similar to those women who experience alcohol as pleasurable, these women are involved in negative drinking. Experiencing negative drinking, they are unable to cope with feelings that come up in their specific social situations as women. For them, to actually feel the emotions that arise in their particular life situations is not allowed. These feelings are experienced as threatening to them and so they will not allow themselves to continue to feel them. They use alcohol to help them to manage their negative feelings. Unlike the women who experience positive drinking and who use alcohol in social situations as a social lubricant, these women use alcohol as a medication. Alcohol becomes a 'cure all' for their personal and social ills. Their medication, alcohol, is self-prescribed. Most important, they have little if any control over this self-chosen antidote, and they experience difficulties with this 'cure'.

Why negative drinking?

If we focus on the reasons why women experience negative drinking, we have a sense, from the examples given above, that something is not right in the lives of these women. Nevertheless, it may be hard for us to put our finger on the problem areas. What we do know is that 'this something' has to do with burdensome or unbearable feelings that are not necessarily shared by other women in similar situations. On some level, women experiencing negative drinking disapprove of their feelings. They are unable to cope with them.

A whole series of feelings have been related to women's negative drinking: boredom, fear, anxiety, stress, sense of loss, guilt, shame, anger, frustration, rejection, despair, loneliness, sense of inferiority and rage.[11] But there may be many more feelings or mixtures of feelings that can be linked to women's negative drinking.

One woman described how her negative drinking began because she felt inadequate as a woman in social situations. She was timid, and this experience of timidity made her fearful of others:

> My abuse of alcohol has to do with my own shyness and fear of other people. I am so shy. Alcohol helped me to cope with being shy.

Women are popularly seen as being a little less confident – more shy – than men. It is considered appropriate for women to be bashful and perhaps even flirtatious with this bashfulness, but they are usually expected to be affable. To be withdrawn is unacceptable.

Pressures can also arise from one's own expectations. One woman describes how for her alcohol became a comfort in an otherwise lonely and isolated life. Alcohol was her only consolation; it was a means of solace. Her use of alcohol had intimate, sexual connotations; alcohol was her lover, her paramour, albeit a secret one.

> I thought the greatest lover in my life was alcohol. It was the be all and end all for me – just like a very close and dependent sexual relationship.

For this woman, alcohol filled a psychological gap in her life. At the time she was overdrinking, she believed that alcohol was helping her to cope with a life that lacked intensity and a passionate relationship. She craved passion and directed hers to alcohol. But, as she recalls, 'the relationship turned abusive'. In expressing her unfulfilled passions through alcohol, she was in fact abusing her longing body and her lonely spirit. Alcohol became a 'lover' who betrayed her.

It is only recently that researchers have looked into links between the use of alcohol and violence that women experience in their actual relationships. Furthermore, while the links between alcohol and violence and their impact on gender relations are being recognised,[12] alcohol has also been seen as an instrument of 'intimate domination'.[13] In other words, alcohol can be intrusive within, have a violent effect upon and exacerbate domineering behaviour in intimate relationships. We already know that any type of violence against women, whether experienced as sexual, physical or psychological, can have a destructive impact on a woman's life. Putting alcohol into the violence-against-women picture will only compound the brutality. Violence may be directed towards women by men who drink too much. Alternatively, women may also themselves become violent if they drink too much. Although this type of violence is less documented than violence against women, it does exist and may be directed towards friends, partners or children.

Women who have experienced physical, psychological or sexual violence and abuse from men may begin to drink too much. Sometimes, a male partner is abusive while the female partner drinks to cope with the abuse. This tends to develop into a cycle of abuse, as one woman described:

> I had been married to someone who used to beat me . . . He was drinking. I did not drink so much in the beginning, but as the abuse got worse so did my drinking and I was drinking to cover my pain . . . It was an endless cycle.

For this woman, the reason she drank was to cope with the pain of physical beatings and abuse from her husband. Alcohol was her antidote, her self-prescribed 'cure' for both the physical and psychological pain she experienced in her particular, intimate situation of domestic violence. While alcohol did not take the physical and psychological pain of abuse away, it did at the very least allow this woman, in her view, to protect herself from feeling the anguish of a situation in which she was trapped. But the irony is that in order to protect herself from the pain of feeling physically and psychologically hurt, she, in turn, abused herself by drinking too much. This is why she saw her situation as an 'endless cycle'. She could not stop.

MASCULINITY, FEMININITY AND ALCOHOL: 'REAL MEN DRINK; NICE GIRLS DON'T'

The gender dynamics of alcohol use in society still need to be uncovered. For example, for women involved in negative drinking, there exists at some level social disapproval and rejection. These women put their femininity and female roles in society at risk. Given that all hear the message, 'Nice girls don't drink too much', women who do drink too much are saying a big 'no' to society. They do that unacceptable thing: lose control.

While alcohol is an integral part of the daily life of a woman who experiences problems with alcohol, it is not a very pleasant one. As we shall see, on the contrary, her life is full of misery. Added to this daily distress is an intense awareness of failure. In drinking too much, a woman is seen to have sacrificed herself to the bottle. In society's eyes, she has failed as a woman. In a real sense, she has lost her womanhood. What is crucial here is that if a man drinks too much, he tends to be seen in an opposite light. His masculinity can be established through a bottle. 'Real men drink' is the message directed to male ears. This message could be interpreted as permission for men to drink more than women.

One woman, reflecting upon her earlier years in college, said:

> I never knew most of my women friends to get drunk like the men did. Most of my women friends just seemed to get sick and tired . . . while the men just seemed to keep drinking and drinking sometimes to the point of passing out.

In a similar vein of thought another woman said:

> I think that when men are drunk it is considered part of the norm . . .

Here, we see that alcohol use may be more linked to gender relations than has previously been considered. Women who overdrink are judged more harshly than men who do likewise. Drinking norms tend to uphold existing gender relations and expectations. As this book will show, on the one hand, men are viewed as the dominant 'actors', encouraged to prove their virility through drink. On the other hand, women are viewed as on the periphery of drinking norms and punished more severely if they drink too much.

THE ECONOMICS OF ALCOHOL USE

As discussed briefly above, there is a general trend in alcohol research to overlook social inequalities based on gender, race, class, sexual orientation, disability, age and so on. Related to this trend is the fact that discussions about the ideological, economic or political importance of alcohol are few and far between.

There is an immense, hidden contradiction which becomes visible when we look closely at this area. As an acceptable social drug, alcohol is encountered on a daily basis: it is advertised on the television, in magazines, on billboards, in public transport systems, in restaurants, in cafés, in bars, in pubs, on cars, on T-shirts, on sport caps and in blinking neon lights. In many ways, alcohol advertising has gone out of control. As one woman aptly states:

[It's as if] alcohol should be everybody's friend . . . It should be a central part of everybody's daily life.

But while bombarded with alcohol advertising and the not-so-hidden message to drink, a woman who drinks too much experiences shame. She is perceived as being weak.

People in western societies tend to spend a lot of money on alcohol. They work hard and at times drink hard – using hard-earned money. For example, in the United Kingdom around 7.5 per cent of all consumer spending is on alcohol;

as a nation, Britain spends about £33 million on alcohol each day.[14] Most governments make huge profits from alcohol taxation. For example, the British government makes approximately £5,000 million a year from taxes on alcohol. Producing, distributing, marketing and consuming alcohol involves huge amounts of money on local, national and international levels. There is a US $170-billion-a-year global alcohol market, dominated by 27 major multinational corporations. Each corporation has sales exceeding US $1 billion a year and branches in eight major industrialised nations. During the economic recession of the late 1970s, many British multinationals sought new markets in developing countries and expanded home markets through alcohol sales in multiple retail chain stores. Alcohol became available at lower retail prices. One major consequence of this development was that women became increasingly targeted by alcohol producers and retailers.

Special products were designed for female consumers. The industry sponsored cocktail bars to attract a female clientele and targeted women through the advertising of exotic drinks directed more towards female than male palates. In addition, it was believed that women's access to alcohol would increase by making alcohol available in supermarkets, which were seen as shopping spaces for women more than men. By the mid-1970s half of Britain's supermarkets had licences to sell alcohol.

In this situation, profit from alcohol consumption appears to take priority over public health – specifically women's health. Any woman suffering from alcohol-related problems is labelled 'an alcoholic' and 'a drunk'; it is her fault if she gives in to the 'temptation to drink'. And yet these beliefs exist regardless of the fact that the messages women receive are to drink and to drink more. In effect, as we shall see, women lose out not only by being prime targets for the aggressive marketing strategies of the alcohol industry but also by appearing to be out of control, a social threat, sexually permissive, destructive and endangering their family's stability and well-being if they overdrink.

One woman who is quite critical of the alcohol industry's marketing strategies believes that the message to continue to drink is one sponsored by 'the distillers and the brewers'. In her view, alcohol abstinence is not even seen as a real possibility in our society. She says:

> Alcohol is really pushed on people. Abstinence is not a viable option. This pushing is sponsored by the distillers and brewers. They say we do not want anyone to stop drinking because then we don't sell our products.

For her, the alcohol industry is the 'pusher' of legal drugs (ie alcohol) in society.

THE METHODS USED IN WRITING THIS BOOK

In unearthing the genealogy of the women and alcohol issue, we need new forms of seeing. Although I am a researcher and a sociologist, I have consistently held that good research and writing must always take the 'view from below' and *make that view visible*. This is really the view from women alcohol users themselves. I use the word 'below' here because that is how traditional work in this area, with very few exceptions, sees women.

I shall attempt to challenge the traditional view on women and alcohol by 'upping' the view from below and making this view most important throughout the book. After all, who knows best about the women and alcohol issue than the women who drink or who have problems with drink? Why do women drink? How does drinking affect our psychic and social lives? What symbols does alcohol use have for us as women? Do we make connections with our bodies when we drink? And how can an understanding of this issue, women and alcohol, help us as women? These are the key questions asked throughout this book. In my work I have heard many answers to these questions from women who drink, and I believe them. Some of my colleagues disregard this and attempt to put their own words into these women's mouths. But listening to women drinkers themselves can be invaluable.

In order to get the best picture possible from women themselves, I present material from discussions and interviews with both women who have problems with alcohol and those who don't. This work has not focused solely on women problem drinkers because the main aim is to examine what alcohol means in our lives, as women, whether or not we have problems. For example, it has been my experience that many women might not have a problem with their own drinking but they may have a partner (whether a woman or man) who does. So alcohol for these women takes on a different meaning. In many ways, they are forced to experience the effects of an alcohol problem. Sometimes, whether they like it or not, these women end up managing another's problem. At other times, alcohol is linked with domestic violence, and here we can ask how do these women cope?

As far as representing different groups of women, I have attempted in this work to look at the issue of difference. It is important for the reader to be aware that if one is a lesbian, a woman of colour or a disabled woman, for example, having an alcohol problem is experienced in a different way both personally and socially than it is by women who are less marginalised.

I would like to make one final point on methodology.

Overall, I believe that developing a women-sensitive methodology in this area implies that one is not judgemental of the women one studies. This should be of primary importance, a guiding principle. The only judgement that one needs to make in this area is that we live in a society that makes drinking and overdrinking more acceptable for men than for women. Women who drink and have problems are seen as stigmatised. They have to face society's judgement and even the wrong judgements of those who treat them – that they are unfeminine, not real women, bad women, bad mothers, etc. It would be unfair and wrong if after reading this book women readers feel terrified every time they lift a glass of alcohol. A women-sensitive perspective need not be prohibitionist. It merely needs to assert that alcohol can be socially useful for women if used in moderation.

THE STRUCTURE OF THIS BOOK

Chapter One, 'Women's use of alcohol', shows how traditional ideas on alcoholism have developed. Here, we will look at the people who have created these ideas, their theories on alcoholism and the problems that have resulted from these ideas. We will see that the needs of women have been constantly hidden in general ideas on alcoholism. In addition, the focus, in the alcohol field, on psychological and physical addiction as well as moral failure has been limited to a search for causes within individuals, with 'individuals' viewed primarily as men or male alcoholics. Alcoholics and alcoholism have been studied mainly from the viewpoint of treaters and experts – not the treated alcoholics themselves. Here, the terms 'addiction dependence' and 'subordination dependence' will become useful as we look more closely at women's use of alcohol. I will also explain why within a women-sensitive perspective, the term 'substance use' is perhaps more important to women than the terms 'disease', 'addiction' and 'illness'. With the aim to develop new ideas, I will look in more detail at the expression 'heart hunger' and 'body hunger'. In the second part of this chapter, these types of women's hunger will be linked to other ideas on women's use of alcohol.

Chapter Two, 'Multiple problems and women's drinking', shows that the problems women experience with alcohol are many. We look at how women drink and the effects on their lives and relationships. Here, focus is on women's experience of negative drinking. Problems become visible physically, emotionally and in women's relationships with others. Factors such as racism, classism, ageism, heterosexism and every other system of inequality that erodes women's power, their courage, their integrity and their self-esteem contribute to women's sometimes complex relationship to alcohol. Negative drinking contradicts social ideals of feminine behaviour. As a result, women experience a multitude of problems (or 'polyproblems'), making them unable to fit comfortably within society.

In Chapter Three, 'Multiple images and social hypocrisy', are discussions of some of the images women encounter when they are drinking either positively or negatively. We shall see very clearly why women's drinking is different from men's. There is no doubt that women problem drinkers present a direct challenge to social stereotypes of normal, acceptable women. Regardless of whether or not we drink, we share the same cultural commandment to be the guardians of moral and social values. While this commandment has been preserved over the ages, women's role has been equated with a type of stabilizing function of wife and mother. Women who overdrink present a special threat to this traditional female role. They are considered to have deserted respectability in every area of their lives. Since there is a greater chance that moral judgements will be made about women who drink excessively than about men who are heavy drinkers, a double standard can be seen to exist in society.

There are well-established stereotypes of drinking women. As the list of stereotypes grows, more women are being stigmatised. Here, we will see why fewer rather than more stereotypical images are needed and, more important, why these images need to be overturned. We will also see how an awareness of the women and alcohol issue should draw attention to current presumptions about pregnant women and alcohol.

Chapter Four, 'Female "treatment" or women-healing?', looks at the traditional idea of female treatment and contrasts it with women-healing. What does treatment mean and how has treatment 'treated' women? In answering these questions, we will move towards a new level of understanding women's healing processes. We will look beyond treatment settings to gain a full view of women – some women do not seek or want treatment. We will see the need to speak about women-helping and women-healing, but this view is a non-traditional view, a view hidden in the alcohol treatment field.

To build a view based on women's needs and experiences is to be aware that treatment as well as overdrinking can damage women. Therefore, we need to discard a view of treatment based on treaters 'in the know' who appear over and above women. By hearing women's words spoken clearly and with compassion, we will begin to learn about the power and hope of healing for women who experience negative drinking.

Chapter Five, 'Becoming strong: women-sensitivity and self-help', looks at the issue of self-help in the alcohol field and the roots of women's involvement in this type of movement. If women are going to heal themselves, they need to allow themselves to become strong. They need to develop strength, regardless of whether or not their ideas of what it means to be strong differ one from another. A study of what makes women strong should allow women who have problems with alcohol to make more choices for themselves but, more important, to know clearly what these choices are.

Chapter Six, 'Mixing women-sensitivity with alcohol: a Molotov cocktail?', examines strategies for change and new approaches to theories about women's drinking. We look at women's alcohol use in the context of stress. We see how women are able to become active in healing and learn to empower themselves. This, the final chapter, is in fact a beginning. By understanding new approaches to theory, we are better able to examine myths and symbols that can be helpful in the healing process for women who overdrink.

Notes

1. I have discussed these ideas in Chapter Two, 'Women and alcohol', in my previous book, *Women and Substance Use* (London: Macmillan and New Brunswick, NJ: Rutgers University Press, 1992) I demonstrated how substance use, including the use of alcohol, is an important part of many women's lives.

2. See Sarah Hafner, *Nice Girls Don't Drink: Stories of Recovery* (New York: Bergin and Garvey, 1992), p.xix.

3. See Dimitra Gefou-Madianou, ed, *Alcohol, Gender and Culture* (New York and London: Routledge, 1992); and Maryon McDonald, ed, *Gender, Drink and Drugs* (Oxford: Berg Publishers, 1994), for recent examples of the social scientific view.

4. An interesting book that looks at the deep symbolic meanings of alcohol for women is Marion Woodman, *Addiction to Perfection: The*

Still Unravished Bride (Toronto: Inner City Books, 1982).

5. At times I use the word 'alcoholic' in this book. I put it in inverted commas because I don't like the word and its negative associations. However, I am aware that for some people it does not have a negative meaning and is used in a neutral way.

6. This is described in Lillian Faderman, *Odd Girls and Twilight Lovers: A History of Lesbian Life in Twentieth-Century America* (New York: Viking Penguin, 1991).

7. See Rosemary Kent, *Say When!: Everything a Woman Needs to Know about Alcohol and Drinking Problems* (London: Sheldon Press, 1990), where she acknowledges that some women do not seek treatment or help from 'outsiders'.

8. These issues have been discussed in the context of British services. For example, see Jan Waterson and Betsy Ettorre, 'Providing Services for Women with Difficulties with Alcohol and Other Drugs: The Current UK Situation as Seen by Women Practitioners, Researchers and Policy Makers in the Field', *Drug and Alcohol Dependence* 24 (1989): 119–25.

9. Here I am making a distinction between 'positive drinking' and 'constructive drinking'. The latter term, developed by anthropologists, refers to the generalised and constructive social rituals around alcohol use in society. See Mary Douglas, ed, *Constructive Drinking: Perspectives on Drink from Anthropology* (Cambridge: Cambridge University Press, 1987).

10. Throughout this book, I will be using the words of women who have discussed with me their use of alcohol. The work presented was not part of an official, funded research study on women and alcohol. Rather, these words came from my own study and observations, lasting from 1978 to 1991. As a woman researcher in the alcohol field, I heard the opinions of approximately 200 women who shared their experiences of and views about alcohol use with me. I recorded these in my work diaries, noting – either verbatim or in summary form – what they had said to me. Some of these women experienced problem drinking and some did not. The majority of these women were those I met doing research or voluntary work in the alcohol field in the UK, USA and Finland. A minority of women were colleagues (ie either treaters or researchers) and a few were friends. The discussion settings included official alcohol treatment centres, non-statutory alcohol agencies, AA meetings, workplaces and women's homes. In 1991, I decided to use a tape recorder to record detailed

discussions with 10 women. My main aim in taping these sessions was to review questions that came up in my earlier discussions with other women. The material used in this book comes from both taped and untaped discussions.

11. See the now classic article by Linda J Beckman, 'Women Alcoholics: A Review of Social and Psychological Studies', *Journal of the Studies of Alcohol* 36 (1975): 797–824. Here she reviews research that attempted to explain the problems women experience with alcohol as well as the reasons why women overdrink.

12. See, for example, JD Atwood and T Randall, 'Domestic Violence: The Role of Alcohol', *Journal of the American Medical Association* 255 (4) (1991) 460–61.

13. See Robin Room, 'Alcohol as an Instrument of Intimate Domination', paper presented to the Society for the Study of Social Problems Annual Meeting, New York, August 1980.

14. For a fuller discussion of this area and more statistics, see Chapter Two, pp 34–6 in Elizabeth Ettorre, *Women and Substance Use*.

CHAPTER 1

Women's use of alcohol

INTRODUCTION

This chapter is about ideas, providing the background for this book and offering a new conceptual framework for understanding women and alcohol. It describes concepts such as substance use, hierarchy of drugs, addiction dependency and subordination dependency, which are helpful in understanding the impact of alcohol on women's lives. How is the alcohol issue linked to women's roles, position and experiences? We will look at 'heart hunger' and 'body hunger' and how these types of hunger can be linked to women's use of alcohol. How have traditional ideas on alcohol and alcoholism been presented? The following discussion uses the words 'alcoholism' or 'alcoholic' rather than 'negative drinking' or 'women who overdrink' in order to bring out some of the problems within these traditional ideas.[1] This chapter will ask the following questions: Who are the people who have created these traditional ideas? What have these people said? And what sorts of problems have resulted from what they have said?

In answering these questions, we remember that alcohol was viewed as an addictive substance in society long before other types of addictive drugs, such as opium or nicotine, became visible. Today, there are many different and conflicting ideas put forward about alcohol and the causes of alcoholism. It seems as if there are as many ideas on why people are dependent on, addicted to or 'hooked on' alcohol as there are people who are alcoholics.

In talking about the many ideas that exist about alcohol and alcohol addiction, one woman who has worked with alcoholics for over 25 years sums it up nicely:

> Every professional seems to have their own theory about alcohol addiction and alcohol use . . . They are quite happy to follow others – say Freud in areas of sexuality or someone else about spirituality . . . But when it comes to addiction everyone has their own views – like it is the fault of society, religion, economics or whatever . . . Everybody has a theory on addiction – everybody – and they are all different.

WHO ARE THE PEOPLE WHO HAVE CREATED THE IDEAS?

Ideas about alcohol, alcoholics and alcoholism have been created by people who over the years have been active in the alcohol field[2] or who, in the words of Katherine van Wormer, have used 'alcoholism as a way of thinking'.[3] Over time, these individuals have included the alcoholics, both men and women, who have experienced problems with their alcohol use; those who may or may not seek treatment; members of Alcoholics Anonymous (AA) or any other non-treatment group set up specifically for alcoholics; members of temperance groups (eg people who want to prohibit alcohol use in society); members of the alcohol trade (eg those in the brewing and distilling industry, or simply the people who market and produce alcohol); alcohol researchers, chemists, biologists, sociologists, historians, psychologists, pathologists, pharmacologists, endocrinologists; government officials and politicians who make the alcohol policies and laws; and treaters including doctors, nurses, social workers, counsellors and psychotherapists.

All of these people have held different ideas about not only why people drink alcohol but why we become dependent upon or addicted to alcohol. The only area of agreement amongst these individuals, regardless of the particular expressions they use (eg 'chronic alcoholism', 'the disease of alcoholism', 'inebriety', 'alcohol addiction', 'drunkenness', 'alcohol dependence', 'problem drinking', and so on), is that alcohol abuse can be a very sure way to destroy any person's life. The field of study is clearly immense. But what have these people said about alcoholism? How do they describe it? Do they look for causes?

WHAT HAVE THESE PEOPLE SAID?

As suggested from the above discussion, there are many different ideas about alcohol use, alcoholics and alcoholism in society. All of these ideas or theories are attempts to understand why some of us drink too much and indeed harm ourselves physically, psychologically and socially through alcohol use. Very often the experts studying alcohol abuse have talked about what they call 'the disease of alcoholism'.[4] For them, this disease can be seen as caused by genetic inheritance; an allergy; an imbalance between different parts of the brain; a brain condition; a vitamin shortage; or a glandular disorder. This disease of alcoholism exposes a physical addiction to alcohol or a biological compulsion to drink. This physical addiction is rooted in some deep physical and hidden area within the body of the alcoholic. In this view, the alcoholic as a diseased person is viewed as having no control over her/his relationship to alcohol. Unlike moderate drinkers, someone afflicted with this disease of alcoholism is unable to drink in a controlled way. Simply, the alcoholic's compulsion to drink is located in a physical defect. The only 'cure' for this affliction is to stop drinking altogether. Here, these experts talk about total abstinence.

Seeing some truth in these above views, members of AA hold to the idea that alcoholism is a gradual or 'progressive' illness over which an alcoholic has no control or power. However, members of AA are not overly concerned with a cause or the causes of the disease of alcoholism. Whether or not they may locate this illness in a bodily defect or deficiency, members of AA emphasise the need for themselves and others outside of AA to see that alcoholics have absolutely no control over their drinking; that the only way to overcome the illness of alcoholism is by not drinking at all (ie total abstinence); and that confirmed (ie 'chronic') alcoholics can learn how to stop drinking from other alcoholics in the supportive environment of AA. The idea behind the AA philosophy is 'once an alcoholic always an alcoholic'. Therefore, the emphasis is on alcohol as being a physically addictive drug, creating a compulsion to drink in all alcoholics.

Besides seeing alcoholism as a disease or a physical addiction, others have talked about alcoholism as being a pathological state or a psychological disorder.[5] For example, the individual alcoholic is viewed as someone who is using alcohol as a drug to heal the pain of growing up; to cope with wounds inflicted during childhood; or to handle intensely felt damage experienced through a broken home, physical or sexual abuse, a bad marriage or any other psychological problem. Here, the emphasis is on what is hidden, 'ill' and breaking down in the personality, the mind or the unconscious rather than on any physical illness or disease located in the body. Other experts, in an attempt to combine the intricate workings of the mind and body, speak about alcoholism as a complex psycho-physiological disorder, connecting the ideas of alcohol addiction as physical and psychological.

Along with psychological ideas, some individuals have put forward the idea that alcoholic drinking is all about learning harmful or bad habits from one's parents, family, friends or in one's environment.[6] This idea emphasises both how we learn to drink as an intricate process and the importance of this learning process in any individual drinker's life. In light of this, the alcoholic is the one who learns to drink badly or in an abusive, harmful way. Within this view, the only way to deal with this bad habit, alcoholism, is to re-learn how to drink alcohol in a less harmful but controlled way.

Still others put forward the idea that alcoholism is at heart the fault of the alcoholic, the one who drinks too much. In some fundamentalist religions, for example, alcoholism is a vice; the person who drinks in an alcoholic way, that is out of control, is wicked. While the alcoholic may be punished by society for behaviour that is perceived as anti-social, she/he is also perceived as being in need of reform or conversion. Even outside such religious belief some individuals argue that alcoholism is a sign of moral weakness – a character flaw manifested in a lack of will power.

WHAT SORTS OF PROBLEMS HAVE RESULTED FROM THESE TRADITIONAL IDEAS?

There are a series of problems that have arisen from the above types of ideas. There are far too many to discuss, so I will confine myself to four of them.

First, the idea that the disease of alcoholism is rooted in a hidden, bodily area such as an alcoholic's genes, brains or glands puts the main focus of alcoholism on a fault in one's body or physical make-up. Accepting this view may imply that having a problem with alcohol is not the responsibility of the individual alcoholic. Simply, one can get away with saying, 'After all, I was born this way', 'I have this disease or progressive illness', and 'I cannot help how much I drink'. If this disease idea is upheld, the blame is placed on 'alcoholics' bodies'. Alcohol and free will are totally written out of this picture.

One woman I spoke to, an alcoholic of 10 years, rejects the idea that alcoholism is rooted in the body or in an inherited disease or is caused by some genetic or glandular malfunction. In her view, the cause of alcoholism is simply alcohol, a physically addictive drug:

> This is where I get myself into trouble with others. So very few people think that maybe alcohol has something to do with addiction. They just do not think that ingesting an alien substance has anything to do with being addicted to alcohol. Very few people think that maybe alcohol has something to do with alcoholism. They think that the alcohol substance is not important.

On the other hand, this woman also believes that if women drink too much and have problems, they need to look into themselves, their hidden selves. She believes that if they really look within, they will find hidden causes for their alcohol problem. These causes are not biological or physiological, as believed by the proponents of the disease idea; rather they are a mixture of the physical, psychological and emotional. This woman believes that she holds a minority view and that her view is not shared by the majority of those active in the field of alcohol:

Some experts go further than those who believe in the disease model. They say there are lots of factors outside of a person that are responsible for drinking – culture, society, religion, whatever you like. But for me I see that the fault lies in ourselves and our emotions.

So, emotional factors and the addictive quality of alcohol will need to be injected into traditional discussions of alcoholism that stress the faulty bodies of alcoholics.

Second, linked with the above problem, many of the explanations of alcoholism focus on the individual person who is the alcoholic. Alcoholism is individualised. Therefore, any alcoholic's difficulties with alcohol tend to be seen as a very specific problem within one's biology, physiology, behaviour, psychology or morality. Most of these approaches focus on individual causes of alcoholism. As a result, these ideas tend to cover up important social factors that could be related in some way to either the cause or the continuation of alcoholism. These factors include social background, income, working conditions, housing, relationships, ethnicity, age, sexual orientation, gender, and so on.

For example, if a woman of colour begins to overdrink regularly because of the stress of her parental responsibilities (ie she has four children around the age of puberty), she may find that she drinks even more when she becomes the target of racism. Another woman of colour may find that her period of overdrinking actually began when she first experienced racist attacks at her workplace. If we were to focus mainly, if not only, on these women's biology, behaviour, or morality, we would lose a valuable insight into the links between alcoholism and racism in these women's lives.

Besides missing out valuable social issues, the focus on the individual person who is the alcoholic props up the professional careers and working interests of those who treat alcoholics. These alcoholics are seen to need specialised, individualised treatment. 'Alcoholics cannot help themselves; they need us' is the chorus from the treaters. More than any other group in the alcohol field, the treaters are given the power to be seen as 'the experts'. It is the treaters, not the alcoholics, neither the women nor the men, who are seen to be in the know. Although it is the alcoholics who experience these problems, their views on how they experience them are often marginalised. Treaters' individualistic focus re-enforces this marginality.

Third, some of the traditional ideas lay unfairly, in my view, heavy moral judgements on alcoholics. Alcoholics are severely stigmatised by the fact that they are seen as being addicted either psychologically or physically to alcohol. Let us look at this more closely. When we are judged as being bad, sinful, immoral or evil by other members of society, we will find it difficult if not impossible to heal ourselves. On the one hand, we will have to deal with the self-righteousness of those who judge us. This brings us shame. We are seen as less good and as irresponsible members of society in comparison to these morally upright others. On the other hand, we will need to deal with the actual guilt of being made to feel bad, evil, wicked, and so on by those accusing us, before we can concentrate on our own problems with alcohol.

Imagine trying to heal ourselves or deal with our own personal problems if we are constantly being told that we are degenerate, wicked or devils in disguise. Neither shame nor guilt is helpful in the healing process. In fact, shame and guilt, in my view, can inflict as much emotional damage as the actual experience of alcoholism itself.

Fourth, all of the traditional ideas on alcoholism focus

mainly, if not solely, on the male alcoholic. What becomes clear as these ideas are produced is the belief that alcoholism is mainly a men's disease or a male problem. The idea is, for example, that 'real men drink'. If women appear in the analysis at all, our problems with alcohol, our issues and our feelings are lumped together with men's. This is often confusing for women and, as we shall see, unhelpful in their healing process.

DEVELOPING THE CONCEPT 'SUBSTANCE USE'

In order to explore fully women's relationship to alcohol, one needs to be attentive to a perceived truth – there are many social complexities that need to be unravelled and that are invisible no matter how closely one looks at this relationship. To some extent, all societies are dependent economically, politically and culturally on a cushioning process. This cushioning process is all about how people deal with unbearable stress in society, and this process is preserved by the legal and illegal sale of a variety of both addictive and non-addictive substances. These substances are seen to act as soothers, consolers and pacifiers – cushions against pain or against what one experiences as difficult emotions.

The fact that this cushioning process exists on such a large scale shows how commonplace it has become to take substances in response to experiences of anxiety, stress and tension. Nevertheless, there is a paradox within this complex social process. Substances, addictive or otherwise, provide only a momentary relief from stress. No substance can resolve the problems of everyday life, and it could be argued that women have more everyday problems due to such factors as their responsibility to look after others and the fact that women are undervalued by society.

The majority of substances that are discussed in the addiction field are mind altering. Thus, experts frequently use the words 'addiction' and 'alcoholism' to emphasise the ability of these substances to 'hook' the user. However, I would argue that these words do not give a clear enough picture of particular problems women encounter with such substances. I believe that the term 'substance use' is more helpful to women than 'disease', 'addiction' and 'illness'. The terms 'substance use' and 'substance users' have different connotations to the terms 'female alcoholism' and 'women alcoholics'. The former do not impose ethical judgements or suggest a moralistic framework, while the latter often do. They are pejorative and used to build images of fallen or morally corrupt women. Women encounter particular, complex problems with substances. More often than not, the harsher way in which women are viewed and treated means that such women are more damaged and debilitated than their male counterparts.

Discussions about women's use of alcohol could benefit from an understanding of women's relationship to food, which for some women develops into another form of substance abuse. Women-sensitive perspectives on food emphasise a specific 'female' problem: many women, regardless of their actual body size, have ambivalent feelings about what they eat. A lot of women develop a problematic relationship to food, while many men don't. Dieting, being afraid of fat and, indeed, a hatred of obesity are all issues that women confront, and they can be agonising. On the one hand, food can be very soothing . On the other hand, it can be 'the enemy', something to be avoided.

The parallels with alcohol are clear — both food and alcohol (as well as other drugs) can be used by women for comfort, but can simultaneously cause them agonising problems, such as guilt and self-disgust. In many studies, food has been linked to a hidden struggle in women for comfort and release from the burdens of femininity.[7] In this struggle, many women grapple with freeing themselves – becoming independent and liberating their bodies from the limitations and constraints put upon them in a society that imposes greater restrictions on their bodies than on men's (demanding, for example, that they be thin, always look attractive, be passive and/or sexually available, don't seriously compete with men in the workplace, and so on). The same could be argued for alcohol use.

This is not meant to imply that a woman experiencing problems with substances has consciously chosen to use these as a quest for freedom. Rather, the aim of this discussion is to show that using substances is a very fundamental but as yet unrecognised part of women's lives and experiences .

Somehow a woman's body is 'not really her own'. From an early age, a woman is taught to be suspicious if not distrustful of her body – it is too fat, too tall, too short, it has to be available to men if they want it. Therefore, is it surprising that some women use substances to reclaim their bodies – to take these bodies back for themselves? Is it surprising that some women want to say this type of 'yes' to themselves? Regardless of the substances a woman ingests, her problems may have more to do with being a woman than meets our eyes. As we shall see, women face a number of particular problems, problems that can stem from male antagonisms and/or are experienced as hatred or dread directed towards them within a masculinist society. And fear can rule the lives of many of these women.

As demonstrated above, 'substance use' is a women-sensitive term. Substance use is also a concept that can provide the needed groundwork for ideas relevant to women. This concept helps us to shift from a predominantly male-oriented to a more female-oriented viewpoint. It provides a gender balance. If an understanding of the women and alcohol issue is to grow, overdrinking women need to unearth their daily experiences. They need to uproot the everyday ordeals that have been buried by traditional misconceptions and distortions about them. Substance use is a valuable concept in understanding women's alcohol use and some of the invisible issues behind this use.

HIERARCHY OF DRUGS

Now let us turn our attention to another concept, the hierarchy of drugs[8] which hints at the ranking of a whole series of drugs in society. These drugs or substances range from good to bad. The good – that is, socially acceptable – drugs are at the top of the hierarchy (eg alcohol and tranquillisers). 'Good drugs' tend to refer to legal drugs. 'Bad' or unacceptable drugs, such as cocaine and heroin, refer to illegal drugs. They tend to be located at the bottom of the hierarchy of drugs.

This hierarchy is dependent on an unequal system of social values as well as primitive ideas of pollution and purity.[9] This hierarchy obviously affects *both* men and women. However, it could be argued that women are put in more socially vulnerable positions than men when they use drugs that are low on this hierarchy. Negative labels are applied to them, and the lower the drug on the hierarchy, the more negative the label.

A close look at the images and social practices of women alcoholics in public and private spaces of their lives reveals how overdrinking challenges traditional female stereotypes and roles related to the identity of a 'real' woman. The female alcoholic in the private area represents femininity misplaced. She has become a symbol of femininity rejected. In the public area, she is perceived as a drunk; one rarely hears her called a drunken woman, or a women drunk – just a drunk. She has become a 'non-woman'. Women are simply not supposed to be on the street, intoxicated, out of control. Her drunken visibility is a direct challenge to the established social order – she should be looking after her home and family, the stereotype tells us, but how can she do this if she is drunk? She is 'prostituting' her identity, and she is as 'low' as a prostitute in society's view, whether or not she is sexually permissive or a prostitute.[10]

Regardless of where women's alcohol use can be located (ie in public or private), a female alcoholic emerges as insufficiently feminine, uncaring about men and risking the loss of male attention and approval. She is viewed as a failure in her sexual identity. She is polluted. As a polluted person, she is seen to reject her identity as a woman: she spoils her identity.

Let us now turn our attention to another concept, dependency.

ADDICTION DEPENDENCY AND SUBORDINATION DEPENDENCY

We need to consider the complexities of the concept of dependency when looking at women's dependence on all sorts of substances, including alcohol. I would suggest that there are two types of dependency – addiction dependency and subordination dependency – which substance-using women experience and which we need to consider.

At a very early age, as many studies have shown, most women learn what it means to become proper, conforming females in a society where men have more privilege and power. Women more than men tend to be socialised into dependency. In the private space of family life, women observe that to be a successful wife and mother means that they need, in some way, to be dependent upon masculinist ways of thinking and upon men and male structures, patronage and authority – otherwise they risk rejection.

But the situation becomes more complex when women overdrink. If women care givers, such as housewives, become dependent on alcohol, many problems emerge when their overdrinking becomes known. A woman may consume alcohol in order to cope with her dependent status of care giver. She may feel bored, frustrated and/or worthless, because the work of housewives is not considered valuable either by the individuals closest to the woman concerned – the husband and children, for example – or by society at large. She will inevitably experience stress as a result of this as well as what can be called a 'dual dependency' problem,[11] a problem relating to both addiction dependency and subordination dependency.

For example, the word 'dependency' comes from the Latin words 'de' and 'pendere', meaning 'to hang from'. In its dictionary definition, dependency has two meanings: 'being reliant on something' and 'being subordinate to'. In this view, there are two social meanings for dependency – one referring to 'addiction' and the other to being 'subordinate'.

The first meaning, addiction dependency, is the unacceptable side of dependency, while the second meaning, subordination dependency, is not only the permissible side of dependency but also the imposed norm for women as a social group. Addiction dependency is socially unacceptable because it is seen to hinder a woman's role, whether this role is as a dutiful wife, a responsible mother, a devoted daughter or a conscientious female worker. On the other hand, subordination dependency is perceived as being socially useful, respectable, highly valued or morally acceptable. For example, the dutiful wife is often dependent on her husband and considered to be less valuable than – subordinate to – him. Her work, for example, is likely to be less respected and/or less well paid. This is the permissible side of dependency and a fundamental part of many women's lives.

In looking at the two sides of dependency, women substance users (eg those who are involved in addiction dependency) can be viewed as female 'losses' in a society that advocates one type of dependency for women – subordination dependency. Ironically, for substance-using women, such as overdrinkers, addiction dependency makes them more often than not dependent upon a male-oriented health care system. Their addiction dependency propels them further into subordination dependency.

Dependency is a complex, multi-dimensional phenomenon for women.[12] Any woman's subordination dependency is all about her being, at the same time, depended upon by others, eg children or elderly relatives. Furthermore, many women depend upon their status as mother, housewife or care giver in the family, and this status is at the core of their identity. A fundamental part of their being dependent women is deep involvement in the social organisation of caring. In dependency, these women find that others (eg family members, significant others and so on) are dependent upon them for their care, whether physical, psychological or emotional. This process creates a cycle of care giving and suggests that women's experience of dependency is different from men's because women's care giving involves this cyclical movement. If these women experience stress (because, perhaps, they are caring for so many people, are working very hard and are feeling pressured, but are also unappreciated), they may eat a little bit too much chocolate, consume a little bit too much food, drink a little too much wine, smoke too many cigarettes, and so on. If addiction dependency develops, their cycle of caring is put into jeopardy.

The main point here is that some women may be propelled into addiction dependency because of their experience of subordination dependency. Addiction dependency is actually framed within this cycle of caring. For whatever reasons, it may be stressful, difficult or even impossible for those women experiencing addiction dependency to become deeply involved in the social organisation of caring. They become dependent on substances such as alcohol because at some level they cannot or do not want to embody the standard role for women – that of dependent care giver.

Objectively, women with a dual dependency problem are seen as failures. Whether single or married, they have failed in their role as dependent care givers by the very fact that they are dependent upon a substance. This substance, whatever it may be, is seen to take them outside of the realm of caring – that realm of the well-established public and private spaces where women should demonstrate feminine caring and, indeed, embody love. Society's view is that if women depend on alcohol (and suffer from addiction dependency) they can no longer be depended upon. They have debased women's role.

A women-sensitive perspective considers these dual meanings of dependency as a key to understanding women's experiences of substances as different from men's. Overdrinking women may need to see clearly the inter-relationship between addiction and subordination dependencies as well as the relationship of both types of dependencies to the public and private spaces of their daily lives. Exposing these inter-relationships shows the importance of the workings of gender and provides a more balanced picture of women's experiences. In other words, women's experiences can no longer be lumped together with men's. This understanding of dependency *vis à vis* women stresses both individual and social factors. It makes the problems of women overdrinkers more visible.

Women overdrinkers may need to develop a collective consciousness of dependency – both addiction and subordination dependencies – in order to close the gap of misunderstanding between their normal selves and addicted selves. They may need to expose collectively both the acceptable and unacceptable faces of dependency. Women's overdrinking needs to become visible because it is not as it appears to be through the lens of society's misconceptions. Alcohol use is or has been a central part of some women's lives. For all women who drink, alcohol use is a 'piece' of their dependency experience.

ALCOHOL AND WOMEN'S HUNGER – EXPLORING NEW IDEAS

In continuing to offer a new conceptual framework for understanding women and alcohol, let us study more closely the concepts body hunger and heart hunger. Body hunger refers to a real physical hunger – a craving which an over-drinking women feels on a physical level, while heart hunger is about her psychological need for alcohol – a need based on her emotions. Here, I will look at how these two hungers can be linked to women's experience of negative drinking.

At first, the words 'body hunger' and 'heart hunger', which I use to explain our dependence on or addiction to alcohol, may appear odd or strange to some readers. This is because these words have not been used before in the alcohol field.[13] Another reason may be that it is difficult for us to imagine that a craving for alcohol can be linked to human hunger. If pictured in our minds, the word 'hunger' calls up the image of a desire for a substance that is actually essential for life, food.[14]

I am using the word 'hunger' here because it emphasises very concretely what some women experience on a continual basis as a deep appetite, a craving for an addictive substance, alcohol. In this way, alcohol can be perceived, like food, as an essential substance in our lives. This appetite can be felt on different levels, including the physical level and the emotional or psychological level. I suggest that these levels can be linked with either body hunger (as in the former level) or heart hunger (as in the latter) and that women experience both hungers in relationship to alcohol.

One woman counsellor[15] who has worked for nearly 15 years with women who have experienced negative drinking, sees both type of hunger in her clients. While she has both male and female clients, she thinks that women's more than men's experiences are misunderstood. For example, she believes that when women feel an urgent need for alcohol it is because we feel something is deeply lacking in our lives – whether psychologically or physically. She says this is never explained in the literature on alcohol. She sees that women crave alcohol because we feel that our bodies and/or our feelings are incomplete without drinking. In her view, women have a physical hunger for alcohol, while they may feel, on the other hand, a type of heart hunger. She links this heart hunger with difficult emotions which cannot be dealt with unless women drink alcohol:

> I use the term 'heart hunger' because a woman's feelings, her emotions, her loves and hates tell her that she needs alcohol. I guess this is similar to what people call psychological addiction. I use 'body hunger' to mean a real bodily need which is felt like a hunger . This is similar to when others talk about physical addiction. I am unable to deny this physical addiction side of alcohol because

that's what women tell me. I think there is a truth to it. Women feel the need for alcohol as a physical need – perhaps as a type of compulsion. This compulsion is different from but linked to the compulsion felt by those who say they are emotionally driven to take a drink to hide their pain. When women talk about their alcohol problems, I hear them talk about these things. I use these terms, heart hunger and body hunger with them and they understand what I mean. These words reflect our lives.

In an attempt to generate greater compassion in our area of study, I focus specifically on the image of the woman alcoholic as a hungry woman, a desperate women and a longing woman. She is a woman feeling empty, but ironically 'full' of despair. Here, we will answer the questions: What are body hunger and heart hunger in relation to negative drinking? And how are these types of hunger experienced by those of us who have problems with our drinking?

Alcohol and women's body hunger – craving and crying out for a drink

In reviewing some of the traditional ideas on alcoholism, we saw that physical addiction meant that an alcoholic experienced a bodily compulsion to drink. As this physical addiction increased, the alcoholic lost control of her/his intake of alcohol. Regardless of the causes of or reasons for this loss of control, alcoholics were seen to physically desire, and indeed crave, alcohol.

Amongst students of alcohol and alcoholism, there have been many debates about whether or not alcohol is really a physically addictive substance. For example, some people, such as psychologists, may emphasise psychological addiction over and above physical addiction. Some may even deny altogether the existence of a physical addiction. Others, weighing the differences between 'nature and nurture' (eg the biology of alcoholism and social facts linked to alcoholism), put their ideas firmly on one or the other side. But, as I hinted at earlier, there exists no firm, scientific proof, on either side, especially when we start looking at causes of alcoholism. It is a very complex issue.

Nevertheless, what we do know is that in comparison to men, women alcoholics experience serious bodily or physiological changes. While we tend to have less body weight than men, we absorb and metabolise alcohol quicker than men. This means that we can drink less than men and yet experience more physical damage. We also do not need to drink as long as men to become alcoholics, and we can experience acute alcohol withdrawal, a withdrawal which can go on for years.[16] All of this knowledge points to the fact that alcohol, taken in excess over long periods of time, has a damaging effect on our bodies[17] and that more often than not, if taken immoderately, alcohol can be experienced as a physically addictive drug for us as women.

One woman, who had been a member of AA for 19 years, spoke about the importance of dealing with alcohol as a drug. She was not overly concerned about the causes of alcoholism or what she called 'the disease model of alcoholism'. For her, alcohol was purely and simply a drug which needed to be dealt with at a very basic level. She believed that AA helped her to face her 'addiction' and to 'gain support from other members'. She says:

> You must deal with the drug in some way. Saying to women 'Well don't take it!' or 'Try to control it' is not really addressing the problem. I think the essential point to make here about why AA is of any use to anybody is because it does provide a type of containment and a

fellowship . . . and you have got women who have been in the same place that you have been and you have got a programme that gives you the means to build up some kind of confidence and . . . ego structure. That is why any arguments that people may have with me about the disease model is irrelevant. Women have got to face the physical addiction side of alcohol.

Another woman, a member of AA and a therapist, also emphasised the need to recognise the physical addiction of alcohol. She believed quite strongly that if this physical side were not recognised, it could cause huge problems. She said:

I sometimes have a problem when I face a female client who has experienced some type of physical, sexual or psychological abuse. Do I counsel the abuse or do I help the woman come to terms with her drink problem? Many women have a physical addiction. Therefore, I think what you need to do is to address the physical addiction in order to build some safe container or strong ego which will be able to face the other problem or contain the other issues. I think we do our female clients a disservice and that it is therapeutic arrogance if we do not face the drinking problem and say, 'Well my client is drinking a lot because she is remembering sexual abuse.' But this is a difficult area.

The above words hint at the idea that regardless of the problems women face, alcoholism is experienced as a physical addiction, a type of body hunger. Simply, alcohol is needed on a bodily level. We crave alcohol. Some female bodies cry out for it.

Here, I prefer to use the term 'body hunger' rather than 'physical addiction', although both expressions mean a physical craving for alcohol. In comparison to physical addiction, body hunger is, in my view, a more hopeful and, perhaps, a more helpful expression for women. Body hunger emphasises the need for us to take responsibility for our consumption of alcohol. Simply, if I say that I am physically addicted to alcohol and can't stop drinking, I could be tempted to give up responsibility to do anything about stopping or reducing my drinking.

For me, the term 'physical addiction' emphasises not only that my body is 'hooked on' this foreign substance but also that alcohol, not me, has overwhelming control over my body. In short, my focus remains outside of myself. If this type of focus is seen as being acceptable, again it may be difficult for me to take responsibility for my drinking and to come off alcohol. On the other hand, 'body hunger' allows for a shift in focus. Rather than looking outside of myself towards this 'liquid substance' drawing me down the slippery slope of addiction, I am now able to see clearly that it is actually me, myself that feels 'alcohol hungry' in my own body and that I am my body.

Alcohol and women's heart hunger – craving for fullness and fulfilment

The views held by a woman who counsels both illegal drug users and alcoholics can help to develop the idea of heart hunger. This woman speaks specifically about women 'coming off' alcohol. She says:

> Women can get off alcohol in many ways. They can do it for themselves. I do not think it is a big thing for women to get off alcohol. There is a whole mystique and lot of myths about women coming off alcohol which are really Hollywood images more than anything . . . But some women have to go to de-tox and hospitals and so on. They may be the really addicted ones. Of course, they find it a

little difficult . . . But, facing life and saying 'yes' to life is
what recovery is all about. But, in spite of that, you come
back to this nothingness. You see that alcohol addiction is
saying a big 'no' to life.

Her words hint at the idea that while body hunger or
physical addiction to alcohol is felt by some if not many of
us, we need, at the same time, to cope with our own
experiences of emptiness, rooted in feelings of being
devalued and unimportant. Here, I would suggest that for us
to learn the reasons why we have said a big 'no' to life is all
about learning to recognise our own heart hunger. It is about
learning how to cultivate a desire to say 'yes' rather than 'no'
to life.

The woman counsellor who spoke earlier in this chapter
distinguished between body hunger and heart hunger. I
think it is important here to discuss her ideas further,
particularly the links she makes in her work between
alcoholism and overeating. She spoke to me about women's
overeating and how she sees these women as 'heart hungry'.
In her eyes, women who overeat experience heart hunger as
a deeply felt longing, grounded in feeling an inner sense of
emptiness and lack of fulfilment. But overeating women
often confuse their heart hunger with real stomach hunger.
She says:

> If you are eating for heart hunger, you can never get the
> feeling that you are full – that your stomach is full. But,
> when you are really eating for the stomach, the physical
> hunger that you feel, you can say after you eat, 'Now I am
> full. I do not want any more.' Eating problems begin
> because you are eating and eating and eating and you
> cannot get what you need because you cannot find
> satisfaction in your life. Your life feels empty.

Similarly, this counsellor sees links between eating disorders and drinking disorders, and she believes that it is healing to recognise heart hunger in both:

> When a woman overeats, she finds that her heart hunger does not satisfy her. She is really not searching for food to be full. Maybe she is searching for a better life, love, to be good enough for someone, a good career, to get rid of anxious feelings. With overdrinking there is the same sort of thing. Most women are overdrinking for those reasons. They may also want to escape something that is anguishing, forget something or look for some comfort in a bottle.

She suggests that we can either use our hurt feelings as an excuse to overdrink or we can learn how to make a difference between what we feel and want and how to express what we feel and want. Although making this difference is not easy for some, it could be a key to drinking moderately. She continues:

> If a woman feels hurt after a working day or when she gets home, she may start to drink . . . But, if she could make a distinction between 'Oh I want to have a good meal and good wine', 'I am thirsty – I would like to have a cold beer' and 'I am hurt', she would not overdrink.

DEVELOPING HEALTHY HUNGER

For many of us who have experienced negative drinking, developing a healthy hunger for alcohol may seem impossible. Indeed, some women who have experienced negative drinking would be well advised to consider stopping drinking altogether – including women who are very seriously dependent upon alcohol (eg who experience withdrawal symptoms such as shaking, sweating, nausea and nervousness after stopping drinking) and women who have medical problems because of their drinking (eg liver damage, pancreatitis, brain damage, etc).[18]

Other women may not have these sorts of problems. Nevertheless, they experience negative drinking and use alcohol as a way of satisfying their heart hunger. For example, they drink as a way of searching for a better life, love, and so on; getting rid of anxious feelings; escaping their anguish or looking for comfort. These women may discover that they can learn to drink positively. Simply, they are able to drink moderately and learn how to develop a healthy hunger for alcohol.

To provide hope and show that it is possible for women who have experienced negative drinking to learn positive drinking, let us refer to the woman who talked about how she had experienced negative drinking when she was a 19-year-old student, attending university. She never experienced withdrawal symptoms or physical damage from her overdrinking, but still she felt that she had experienced negative drinking. At that time, she drank heavily for about four years to cover up her feelings of loneliness. She is 35 years old now and sees herself as a moderate drinker, drinking only on weekends. What is worthy of notice for us here is that this particular woman has interesting things to say about her own body and heart hunger. She makes a link between what she calls 'her hunger for chocolate' and 'her hunger for alcohol':

> I can have a hunger for alcohol like I have a hunger for some foods – let's say chocolates. What is so bad about it? Once in a while even though I do not like chocolates or ice-cream so much – they are just extra things in the world – sometimes I just want them. For instance, sometimes it

just depends upon the weather, my energy or my vitamin C level. Once in a while I just want the taste of chocolate. So maybe my friends or colleagues will say, 'You need something sweet and you should go to the store and buy fruit.' But, I do not want to do that – I just want chocolate. So I think it is the same to have chocolates, a beer or a glass of wine in that way. It is very normal. You just want to have it and your body says so. It is as simple as that. I need a bit of pleasure to feel good.

In contrast to her earlier experience of negative drinking (ie her hunger for alcohol), this woman's hunger for alcohol as well as chocolates appears now to be based on her need for pleasure and wanting to feel good. She is a clear example of a woman who has experienced negative drinking now learning positive drinking. Simply, this particular woman learned how to make a difference between what she feels and wants and how to express what she feels and wants.

The main point here is that she can now concentrate on, as well as feel, a healthy body hunger for whatever substance she desires. She can take these substances inside herself because her heart hunger has been satisfied. But, her focus has shifted from outer substances to her own inner resources, from those 'extra things in the world' to what her body says and, most important, how she feels. To me, this woman's experience is very hopeful.

In this chapter I have attempted to develop new ideas on women's use of alcohol. I have reviewed traditional ideas on alcoholism and their presentation in society, and I have looked at the types of problems created by these ideas. I have explored some of the ways in which these traditional ideas have had a negative impact on us as women, and have begun to develop new approaches to the subject. Most important,

I have looked at heart hunger and body hunger and how these types of hunger can be linked to our use of alcohol. Let us hear the words of a woman who experienced negative drinking for 10 years. Because she had been seriously dependent upon alcohol, she stopped drinking altogether. In talking with her, I somehow had a deep sense that this woman had learned through much pain and suffering how to satisfy a positive heart hunger without drinking alcohol:

> Often in life, we repress the best of us as well as the worst of us. You see this is how we train ourselves as women. If you do listen to your intuition, you let whatever makes your heart sing, sing. Sometimes, that means you have to change your life completely. And of course most of us do not want to do that. But now I say, let us embrace life and not let it pull us down.

Notes

1. People who study alcohol talk about 'problem drinkers' or 'problem drinking'. Some prefer to use these terms rather than 'alcoholic' or 'alcoholism'. These newer terms, 'problem drinkers' and 'problem drinking', are often seen as the best choice of words in order to move away from moral judgements of people who drink too much. I have already discussed my difficulties with using the word 'alcoholic' and the moral judgement its use conveys.

    In this context, I will not use 'problem drinkers' and 'problem drinking' because in my view they refer more to men than to women, regardless of whether or not these terms appear less moralistic.

    The traditional terms 'alcoholic' and 'alcoholism' also refer more to men than women, but I will in this chapter use these more traditional words. This is because they are not only more descriptive but also allow us to see more clearly the sorts of problems that have emerged with the development of traditional ideas.

2. Here, I use the term 'alcohol field' in the widest sense. This expression refers to the area of study in which people connected to or concerned about the use of alcohol in society have been developing ideas for at least the last 300 years.

3. See Katherine van Wormer, *Alcoholism Treatment: A Social Work Perspective*, (Chicago: Nelson Hall Publishers, 1995), especially pp 109–41, Chapter 5, 'Alcoholism as a way of thinking'.

4. The classic book on this topic is E M Jellinek, *The Disease Concept of Alcoholism*, (New Haven, CT: College and University Press in association with Hillhouse Press, 1960) .

5. See Wilfred E Boothroyd, 'Nature and Development of Alcoholism in Women' in Orian Josseau Kalant, ed, *Research Advance in Alcohol and Drug Problems, Volume 5, Alcohol and Drug Problems in Women* (London and New York: Plenum Press, 1980), pp 299–329. In this research review, Boothroyd shows some of the damaging effects of taking an overly pathological view, although he maintains this type of focus himself.

6. A contemporary translation of these ideas can be found in those who uphold theories of co-dependency. See, for example, Jeffrey McIntyre, 'Reflections on Male Codependency' in Claudia Bepko, ed, *Feminism and Addiction* (New York, London, and Sydney: The Haworth Press, 1991), pp 211–24. McIntyre gives an interesting 'twist' by looking at this learning process for men.

7. See, for example, Susie Orbach's classic, *Fat Is a Feminist Issue* (London: Hamlyn Publications, 1978) and her *Hunger Strike* (London: Faber and Faber, 1986); Lisa Schoenfield and Barb Wieser, eds, *Shadow on a Tightrope: Writings by Women on Fat Oppression* (Iowa City, IA: Aunt Lute Book Company, 1983); and Shelly Bovey, *Being Fat Is not a Sin* (London: Pandora, 1989) as examples of work by women in this area.

8. See my earlier work, Elizabeth Ettorre, *Women and Substance Use* (London: Macmillan and New Brunswick, NJ: Rutgers University Press, 1992) for a more detailed discussion of this concept.

9. Mary Douglas in her book *Purity and Danger: An Analysis of Pollution and Taboo* (London and Henley: Routledge and Kegan Paul, 1966) exposes how pollution and purity are fundamental, primitive issues embedded in all societies. In this context, drugs can be seen as polluting substances. The substance user is no longer pure. Purity is valued highly, pollution the opposite, so in this view the user is degraded.

10. In Chapter Two, 'Multiple problems and women's drinking', we will see some of the problems and effects of alcohol upon prostitutes' lives.

11. See Elizabeth Ettorre, *Women and Substance Use*, for a related discussion of this concept.

12. Hilary Graham's work in this area has contributed much to an understanding of women's 'caring' and dependency. Her article 'The Concept of Caring in Feminist Research: The Case of Domestic Service', *Sociology* 25 (1): 61–78, is a good example of this type of work. Another more contemporary twist to this idea can be found in Hilary Rose's *Love, Power and Knowledge* (Cambridge: Polity Press, 1994), when she discusses how women's lives have been framed by 'thinking from caring'. See particularly Chapter Two, 'Thinking from caring: feminism's construction of a responsible rationality', pp 28–50.

13. I first heard the terms 'heart hunger' and 'body hunger' used in a women and alcohol context in a discussion with Irmeli Laitinen, a psychotherapist at the Women's Therapy Centre, Helsinki, in 1993. She noted that these expressions have been used in developing ideas on women and food and that 'hunger' is a powerful word for women. For examples of hunger used in the context of women's overeating, see Kim Chernin, *The Hungry Self: Women, Eating and Identity* (London: Virago, 1985): and JR Hirschmann and CH Munter, *Overcoming Overeating* (New York: Fawcett Columbine, 1988).

14. But we must remember that alcohol is also a food. This point comes out clearly in the works included in Dimitra Gefou-Madianou, ed, *Alcohol, Gender and Culture* (New York and London: Routledge, 1992).

15. Irmeli Laitinen, Women's Therapy Centre, Helsinki.

16. For an interesting discussion of these findings, see JL Forth-Finegan, 'Sugar and Spice and Everything Nice: Gender Socialization and Women's Addiction – A Literature Review' in Claudia Bepko, ed, *Feminism and Addiction*, pp 19–48.

17. We will discuss ideas about the potential damage of alcohol on pregnant women in Chapter Three, 'Multiple images and social hypocrisy'.

18. For further practical information in this area, see Rosemary Kent, *Say When!: Everything a Woman Needs to Know about Alcohol and Drinking Problems* (London: Sheldon Press, 1990).

CHAPTER 2

Multiple problems and women's drinking

ENCOUNTERING BASIC PROBLEMS OF LIVING

For a lot of women, the alcohol substance in that forbidden bottle has become their friend. This is because they are terrified of social situations and thus, alcohol is experienced as a confidant. Of course, these women could easily, perhaps, put a mask on their faces, go out in public, and be polite, but they are petrified of meeting people. They may have poor social skills . . . They are quite frightened and the only way they know how to deal with their fear of social situations is with alcohol – to drink. In their eyes, alcohol is their only true friend.

These words, spoken by a woman who experienced negative drinking for many years, suggest that many women who overdrink often experience problems in relating to others. Their inability to control their alcohol intake is a big problem, but they also encounter basic problems in living. Their difficult relationship with alcohol means that living their everyday lives requires overcoming many obstacles.

In the introductory chapter, we saw that women who are dependent upon alcohol and experience negative drinking do so for a variety of reasons. In this chapter, we will look at these women and see the sorts of difficulties they face in their lives. First, we will look at how the combination of women and alcohol may cause multiple problems for them. Then we will consider three problem areas that become most visible when we look closely at women who drink too much. We will go on to see how women's problems become compounded by social prejudices towards race, ethnicity, age, sexual orientation, disability and so on. Last, we will look at what I have identified as special groups of women drinkers.

MULTIPLE PROBLEMS

'Multiple problems' (or 'polyproblems'[1]) describes the kinds of difficulties and dilemmas that not only become visible in the lives of women who drink too much but also are experienced by them at deep levels. For any woman, a life centred on alcohol is full of these multiple problems in both her private and public life. Whether she is alone at home or out in public, the woman alcoholic's life can be riddled with what has been called 'internalised shame'.[2] The more she becomes psychologically or physically dependent upon alcohol, the more difficult it is for her to remove these problems and to face herself without shame. (This issue will be discussed in more detail later in this chapter.) The problems of women who drink too much differ from the problems of men who drink too much,[3] and social expectations around the use of alcohol are different for women in comparison to men: they are gendered.[4] If a woman does not live up to these social expectations, she might experience conflicts within herself, and these conflicts will differ from men's. The different social expectations around alcohol use as well as the experience of different problems for men and women who drink too much tend to remain hidden in society. Nevertheless, the multitude of problems women encounter because of their use of alcohol can make them unable to fit comfortably within society.

But what are the sorts of problems that women who drink too much experience? In answering this question, we need to focus on areas where women's problems emerge most clearly. In my view, there are three problem areas that become most visible: women's relationship to their bodies, the development of their emotional lives, and their relationship to others.

Alcohol and women's bodies

While we are often presented with glamorous images of a woman with an alcoholic drink in her hand, the actual bodily effects of this substance, if abused, can be less than glamorous. Before discussing the bodily effects, let us ask ourselves the question, What is alcohol?'.

The key issue to remember here is that alcohol is a drug, albeit a socially accepted and legally distributed one. Alcohol is also a psychotropic drug, which means that it has an effect on the mind. It also has physical effects on the body.[5] The alcohol we drink is made from ethyl alcohol, the chemical components of carbon, hydrogen and oxygen. What we drink has been fermented by yeast of sugars that occur naturally in plants. Alcoholic drinks produced by this fermentation, such as beer from barley, wine from grapes and cider from apples, can be weak in alcohol. For example, beer can have between 2.5 and 8 per cent alcohol by volume (that is, only 2.5 to 8 per cent of the total liquid in the bottle is actually alcohol). On the other hand, the concentration of alcohol in spirits is increased by a process of distillation. For example, 40 per cent of alcohol by volume is the usual strength for gin.

Women who drink, both those who drink too much and those who drink moderately, tend to be aware of the physical effects of alcohol on their bodies. These effects range from a mild sense of intoxication to serious physical damage, such as cirrhosis of the liver[6] or brain damage.[7]

When I spoke with women about their drinking, I found that many were particularly aware of the mild, physical effects of alcohol. For example, one woman, reflecting on her earliest experiences of social drinking, spoke of alcohol as 'an elegant part' of her life as well as having 'nice' effects:

> Yes, alcohol can be very glamorous. After drinking it, you begin to know the nice feeling that you can have after a few drinks . . .

Another woman thinks of alcohol as a type of refreshment. It rejuvenates her:

> I like the feeling of a cold beer on a hot summer's afternoon . . . It is so refreshing . . . I feel rejuvenated.

Another woman talked about how, if she made a decision to drink, her experiences of alcohol enhanced how she was feeling in particular social situations. She liked the warm, friendly feelings that alcohol gave her:

> I usually make a decision to take a drink or not to take a drink. Usually when I am with others, say at a party or with close friends, I drink because I like the way my feelings come up with alcohol. These sensations help me to feel warm towards my friends.

As we see from these comments, regardless of the amount of alcohol we drink, alcohol affects the body, often in ways that make us feel good. But because alcohol is a drug, it can lead to dependency. Similar to heroin, tranquillisers, amphetamines or cocaine, alcohol not only produces changes in behaviour and feelings but also has the potential to lead to addiction. Although many women may be aware of the physical effects of alcohol, they may be unaware of the addictive properties of alcohol or the possibility of becoming dependent on alcohol. Often women with experiences of negative drinking do not see themselves as 'addicted' or recognise that alcohol dominates their lives.[8] Some think 'I am not an "addict"'. For them, an addict is an illegal drug user, like a heroin user who will do anything for a 'fix'. It is as if the hierarchy ranging from acceptable to unacceptable drugs, which was mentioned in the previous chapter, is firmly in their minds. While both stereotypes of alcoholics and addicts[9] are negative in society, the image of the woman alcoholic may appear to be less bad than that of the woman addict because she is dependent upon a legal drug. Nevertheless, the physical or bodily damage a woman alcoholic may have in comparison to a woman heroin addict may in some instances be worse.[10]

The physiological effects of alcohol are immense. Alcohol can affect the brain, liver, stomach, intestines, pancreas, heart and blood circulation. The physical problems that women who drink too much experience may include memory loss, blackouts, premature ageing, chronic coughing, malnutrition, heart problems, 'the shakes', tingling in one's toes or fingers, skin problems, liver damage, ulcers and kidney problems.

I remember a very vivid interview I had with a woman who was seriously ill with liver cirrhosis. She told me that she might die in the near future, although her doctor's prognosis was not as pessimistic as hers. She had abused alcohol for a number of years and, as she said, 'I could drink anyone under the table.' Her abuse of alcohol took a real toll on her body and she felt she had to stop. But although she wanted to stop, she felt she needed a drug in her life. Her husband had divorced her and she was now a poor, single parent. It was difficult for her to cope with her feelings of despair.

Before the doctor discovered her liver cirrhosis, she made a conscious decision to stop using alcohol. As a substitute, she turned to heroin, an illegal drug. 'On heroin' her life became difficult to manage. She could not cope with the 'illegal drug scene' and she sought treatment. It was during her treatment as an out-patient at the drug clinic that she discovered she had cirrhosis:

> My drinking . . . yeah it was serious. I drank a lot. I never knew that it would hurt me so much. I guess people think that heroin is the real killer. I tell them just look at me. Alcohol nearly did me in. It may still . . .

One experienced social worker[11] notes that 'excessive alcohol use can shorten the lives of women alcoholics by 10 to 12 years on average'. This researcher also notes that 'death may result through car accidents, overdoses, homicide, suicide, falls, polydrug abuse and drowning'. Whichever way we look at it, excessive alcohol consumption has the impact of a toxic substance on the body, with the added effect of a link to high-risk behaviour.

Some women alcoholics try to keep these physical problems secret. For example, Lucy, one of Sarah Hafner's[12] respondents, spoke, during her story of recovery, of how she was able to 'fool everybody' and how everyone around her 'thought she was functioning', even though she had a severe vodka dependency problem at the time. Nevertheless, these problems can eventually become visible to those near to these women. The effects of their excessive drinking can be observed in their manners, by their movements or in their faces.

One woman recalled her vivid experience of working with

a colleague who was 'alcoholic'. She knew her colleague had a drinking problem, even though this colleague tried to be discreet. She recalls:

> We just knew [she] . . . was really an alcoholic. You just needed to look at her to see it. I know she tried to hide it, by pretending nothing happened, but you could just smell it. Her face was purple. . . .

Alcohol and women's emotional lives

As we have seen from the above, alcohol can have physiological effects upon the body. However, there is no doubt that negative drinking will also have a powerful, if not deleterious, effect upon women's emotional lives. We saw earlier, in the introduction, a whole series of reasons why women experience negative drinking. These reasons more often than not were related to how women felt about themselves. Feelings of inadequacy, loneliness and fear appeared to emerge as key features in these women's emotional lives.

Women who drink too much tend to have a hard time confronting their emotional problems head on. It is also hard for them to understand, as well as to deal with, all sorts of emotions, resulting from powerful social stereotypes, whether self-imposed or imposed on them by others. Stereotypes make it doubly difficult for them to uncover their burdensome emotions.

Related to this, the idea that in comparison to men, women are taught to be the carriers of emotions in society remains visible in the alcohol treatment field.[13] Alongside this is the notion that women who drink too much are 'emotionally crippled'. Of course, men are described similarly. But to describe women as emotional cripples has specific implications for them in comparison to men. When we take into account the fact that women, regardless of whether or not they drink, tend to be socialised into being the carriers of emotions in society,[14] then we realise that being described as emotional cripples is more stigmatising for women. They, more than men, are expected to live up to the social expectation to shoulder feelings and emotions, so they more than men are perceived to have failed. (Of course the term 'emotional cripple' is also an attack on anyone who is in fact physically disabled. It is a derogatory term, suggesting inadequacy.)

In alcohol literature, we are told that women overdrink because they are unable to cope with their feelings of inadequacy, loneliness, frustration and depression.[15] Although this may be true for many women who overdrink, it does suggest a view that feelings, particularly negative feelings, are difficult for every woman who drinks too much.

When a woman is drunk or has been consistently drinking too much, you may hear the expressions 'she's in denial', 'she can't cope with her feelings', 'she can't face herself', 'she can't take it', 'she's bombed out', 'she is comatosed'. These comments suggest a lack of feelings or a pushing away of feelings and imply that she does not value her feelings. In other words, she has emotions, but she would rather be without them. Here, I suggest an alternative view: for any woman who drinks too much, her feelings and her emotions are of the utmost importance. She is very much with her emotions, whatever these may be. If her feelings and emotions are not important to her, why would she go to such extremes (ie overdrinking) to cover them up?

The key issue here is that feelings are valued, but they may be experienced as threatening or unbearable. There is a world of difference between giving feelings importance in one's life and finding one's own feelings threatening. Since, as discussed above, women more than men are supposed to be the 'experts' on an emotional level, this can be experienced as more of a failing in women than in men. But why should women have that sort of social responsibility? It should be quite realistic nowadays to demand that both men and women share the responsibility to be carers and indeed carriers of emotions.

Within this alternative view, it could be assumed that women overdrink, drug themselves with alcohol or self-medicate because they refuse to experience themselves as those in society who can cope easily with emotions. While these women say 'yes' to alcohol, they may be saying a very big 'no' to being chosen as the emotional carriers, carers or copers. But saying 'no' in this way can generate humiliation, feelings of powerlessness, disgrace, self-pity, alienation, depression and, most important, shame.

With regard to this last feeling, one author[16] suggests that in our society shame, as a pattern of mood or feeling, is gender related and tends to characterise women more than men – ie that women are more prone to experience shame and that shame has a different meaning in relation to their personal and private lives than has a similar emotion experienced by men. Furthermore, the experience of shame is compounded when a woman drinks too much.

One woman I spoke to reflected upon her own life experiences and the shame that she had felt from drinking too much. For her, shame was an overwhelming emotion:

> . . . shame is the underlying sort of theme you see going through all of my drinking . . . Shame is not just behind it, but shame is going through it – all of it . . .

For the woman who drinks too much, feelings of humiliation, disgrace, and regret colour all of her experiences on a day-to-day level, but shame is a most central emotion in these experiences. Another woman spoke about how her 'alcoholic' friend's life was filled with disrepute and shame.

As she described her friend, it was almost as if her friend oozed shame in her every movement:

> Everything becomes shameful for [her]. She thinks her behaviour is shameful. She thinks she is shameful. Why? She says she's a mother of three children, a housewife. But she is a shameful drinker . . . She is just a slave to all these people and even that is shameful, too.

Shame is profoundly disempowering for women.[17] In order to overcome their shame, women who experience negative drinking need to know why they have been made to feel shameful and, more important, their 'alcoholic shame' must be confronted.

One woman recalled the power of shame in the lives of all of the overdrinking women she knew. Although, in her view, these women experience a deep sense of shame, they needed to expose shame for what it was — a 'phantom feeling', plaguing them unnecessarily:

> Whatever these women's stereotypes and conditioning, they have been made to feel ashamed about it all . . . Women who are more secret, more hidden and private about their drinking need to get their shame out in the open. They need to admit that they are ashamed and to understand that there is nothing to be ashamed of. Shame is a ghost.

When a woman drinker is seen as failing to be a good mother, being visibly drunk or out of control, she needs to know that she has nothing to feel ashamed of. It is not her fault. At the same time, she needs to uncover other emotions such as guilt, helplessness, despair and fear, which are closely related to her 'internalised shame'. Only when they are recognised and out in the open will she begin to be able to deal with them.

Alcohol and women's relationships

As we have seen, alcohol can have a powerful effect on women's emotional lives and in turn, their relationships to themselves. But negative drinking will inevitably influence a woman's relationships with others. Even if she is able successfully to hide the fact that she overdrinks, she will find that her drinking will affect, in some way, her relationships with her friends, her partner, her husband, her family and/or her workmates. Negative drinking will also bring out a whole series of feelings and behaviours from others. While these feelings may include anger, contempt, disgust, pity and empathy, responses may range from silence, criticism and advice-giving, to outright rejection.

One woman recalled how she worked with a woman who drank quite heavily. She said she remembered the experience 'distinctly'. While she and her workmates remained silent about their colleague's drinking problem, they tended also to protect this colleague:

> People covered for her, I noticed. We – and I say we because there was a group of us, I did it too – we really protected her – covered up for her – and we tried to help her to do her work because we felt sorry for her.

Her colleagues' responses of pity and the need to protect her allowed this overdrinking woman to function, although not well, at her workplace. Other women, not experiencing this type of protection or 'covering up', may find their jobs or livelihoods at risk. If anger or contempt from colleagues is directed towards her and, furthermore, become a destructive influence at her workplace, there is the constant risk that she will lose her job.

Let us look at friendships. I start with the example of one woman of colour who had been drinking heavily for a number of months after she had changed jobs. She moved to a job that was quite demanding and in which she became the focus of much public attention. She had moved very rapidly up the salary scale from a low-paying, menial job to a higher-paying, senior administrative job for which she was very qualified. But the work was demanding much of her time in the evenings and at weekends. She started drinking socially to cope with the stress of her new job. But when she drank she became aggressive and spoke abusively towards her friends and colleagues. Sometimes, as she recalls, she could not remember what happened after she had been drinking all evening:

> I cannot remember when it hit me . . . [name of friend] told me to shut up and cool down. She told me if I didn't wise up, [name of another friend] would go home. I remember we were all at a local pub. I said to myself, yeah cool down, it's easy to say. But, then, I knew I needed my friends. So I stopped drinking for a month to cool down.

This woman's experience of her friend's anger mixed with the threat of possible rejection allowed her to reassess her drinking and to stop drinking excessively at least for a while.

One woman recalled how she used to have a good school friend with whom she drank. At university, they often got drunk together. Over time she drank less, while her friend continued to overdrink. Gradually her friend became out of control at parties and in social situations. She told her friend that if she did not control her drinking, they could not be friends any longer. At first, her friend did not take her advice. She refused to stop drinking and became even more drunk and destructive in social situations. The woman stopped seeing her friend and avoided occasions where she was present. Eventually, a few years later, this friend joined AA. But, in this woman's view, it was too late. Their friendship had not survived. Now they seldom see each other and are no longer friends:

> I never knew what to do when she got drunk. It was OK at university. It was almost expected, but after that and over the years, she just got boring. She never kept her plans with me because of drinking. We always knew if you invite [name of friend] to a party, she would get drunk. One day I just told her that she has a problem with alcohol and why didn't she get some help. I could not help her. I did not see her anymore as a friend. You could not talk with her. Once in a while she calls me, but then all she talks about is AA.

She tried to show empathy and give advice; nevertheless, the friendship was lost. By becoming the central part of this woman's life, alcohol had destroyed a once close friendship.

Besides giving 'free advice', friends, partners or relatives often feel helpless or powerless in the face of a woman who overdrinks. They become aware that to get a friend, relative or partner to stop or at least reduce their drinking is not possible unless the person herself takes control of her own life. It is imperative that she find the power within herself to stop drinking, whether or not she is aware of this fact herself. Often she isn't because she is in a state of active denial. She needs people around her who can be respectful of her and her drinking problem, while at the same time challenge her active denial.[18] If this doesn't happen she won't change. Perhaps she will go on isolating herself, endangering her job, losing touch with friends and forgetting about the need to have good feelings about herself.

When women are 'secret drinkers', these issues become more complex. Usually, secret drinkers sense or know unconsciously that they are involved in destructive drinking, regardless of their level of active denial. But their drinking is a well-kept secret, hidden from others, whether these others be family, friends, relatives, spouses or partners. That their lives revolve around alcohol is their own 'special secret'. They refuse to allow their use of alcohol to become visible to others. Alcohol becomes a type of contraband, similar to goods imported, possessed and used illegally. But, at the same time, alcohol in the form of their special brand of intoxicating substance such as gin, cocktails, beer, whisky, vodka, etc fills the privacy of their own emotional lives. Visible use of their contraband is a taboo.

In some ways, these women can be likened to smugglers. They become smugglers sneaking alcohol into the private domain: the home. Most important, these female smugglers feel ashamed, guilty or afraid that their secret will be revealed or their 'piracy' unveiled. For these women, their only hope of survival is to have a clandestine relationship to alcohol.

Women who are secret drinkers not only hide their dependence on alcohol from others but also develop a repertoire, a series of hidden skills, which they use to maintain their secret. For example, there is the compulsory brushing of teeth (usually with strong-smelling toothpaste) or the statutory use of a hardy mouthwash before the husband or children come home, before meeting friends or before going to work. In a pocket or a handbag, there is the need to carry a packet of potent mints, a small can of breath freshener or at least some chewing gum to use wherever one goes – just in case one has a 'quick one' at the local or not-so-local bar, pub, café or restaurant.

Also, there is the need to place one's substance in a 'safe' and out-of-the-way place so that others will not find out one's secret: perhaps hiding one's contraband in a laundry cupboard, in the back garden, in the trunk of the car, with this year's preserves in the basement, behind the sewing machine, etc. For women with fewer luxuries, hiding one's stash in a coat pocket, the shopping bag, the bicycle bag, the motorbike box, the box of old newspapers or under the sink may suffice. Other alternatives may include a nicely decorated silver, bronze, leather or plastic flask, tucked neatly away in one's handbag: 'Oh well, it could always pass as a "female accoutrement" if anyone besides me happens to see it.' Often one's hiding place will be successfully chosen and will be left undiscovered by others for many months or, in some cases, years.

One woman who hid her alcohol in her bedroom for five years recalled her experiences:

> I can retreat into the solitude of my bedroom with my bottle. I can get all dressed up and come out and go to work and do the duties around the house. I can be a mother and drive all of the kids to school and then after work, I can come home and top up. Alcohol is my secret . . .

Another woman, once a secret drinker, relates to the experiences of other women, similar to herself:

> . . . Women drink secretly because women are taught not to get visibly drunk in society . . . they drink alone. They somehow manage to carry on a lot of household duties without a lot of people knowing that they drink. In fact, no one knows. It is strictly hidden. So a lot of the stigma and shame is self-generated.

Besides secret drinkers, there are also women whose problems with alcohol may be less than secret. In other words, these women may have confided in family, friends and relatives, partners or spouses about their use of alcohol. Still, they continue to overdrink. Outside of a close circle of friends, most people they meet will not be aware of their overdrinking. Nevertheless, these women may experience problems with others in a variety of ways. This is because others become involved in hiding their secret or covering for them. Let us look at a series of examples:

Perhaps this woman goes to a party one night and, surprising herself and her accompanying friend, partner or spouse, she actually drinks in moderation. (Before the party, her friend, partner or spouse had warned her that she would walk home if she became drunk. The party was on the other side of the city.) But, upon her return home with her friend, partner or spouse, she decides to continue drinking on her own and downs a bottle and a half of Scotch. After drinking such a large amount of alcohol, she is not only feeling quite ill but is unfit for work the following morning. Her partner, friend or spouse rings her workplace to say that she has flu and will be off from work. This is the fourth time this month that this sort of thing has happened. The partner, friend or spouse is deeply perturbed.

Perhaps this woman is a journalist. She spends one weekday during her working week at home. She likes to work at home. There, she can work in peace and away from the hustle and bustle of the office. But when at home, she drinks alcohol, preferably strong beer. Right now, she needs to complete an article on the changing social life in the community for the local newspaper. In fact, this evening, she has planned to go with friends to an event at the local community club. In her article, she plans to include a small discussion of this event. One of her favourite local poets will be reading her poetry, and soft drinks (ie non-alcoholic) will be served. Before she knows it, it is early evening, and she has been consuming a number of bottles of strong beer all day to 'help her to concentrate'. She realises that she is unable to get herself dressed and ready for the evening's event. Her friends arrive to accompany her, but she explains with much embarrassment that she cannot go; she is too drunk. At this stage, she is unable to stand up — let alone walk. She asks one of her friends to ring the local organisers to say that she cannot go, that she is sorry and that something has come up. 'Give any excuse – any excuse will do', she tells her friend. 'Yes, thank you, I am sure her father will be fine', she hears her friend say over the phone. One of her friends leaves in disgust and slams the door behind him, muttering, 'I cannot stand all of these lies.'

Women who experience overdrinking can become very skilled in the art of deception. There is a tendency, as we see from the examples above, for these women to draw others around them into this circle or ring of deception. By using the strong word 'deception' I am not meaning to suggest that these women are in any way evil, corrupt or degenerate.[19] I use the word to illustrate that more often than not duplicity and falsehood may be an integral part of the lives of women who overdrink. No one, male or female, who experiences negative drinking wants to publicise this fact. It is the rare person who is able to appear publicly, for example on national television, to declare they are an 'alcoholic' or even drunk more often than sober. Why should they?[20] If made visible in public, this type of behaviour is still stigmatised, especially for women. One researcher[21] suggests:

> Stigma remains a very serious issue for women who are alcoholic or addicted in this society. Regardless of social changes in the past 20 years, women are still measured by subtle and pervasive gender norms.

What woman wants to endure more guilt, shame and disgust, if not outright rejection, as a result of being sincere in public? Therefore, it is quite natural that a woman who overdrinks, and those around her, would want to hide this fact from public view. As loyal and faithful friends, partners or spouses, these individuals collude with her in keeping her secret. The irony is that by being loyal, these significant others become very closely involved in this ring of deception.

A friend's, partner's or spouse's loyalty mixed with collusion, deception and secrecy may be perceived as being necessary at certain times – merely for the woman's survival. These types of strategies help to ensure that the boundary of this ring of deception is closed. This boundary needs to be fastened because these significant others know the woman has a lot at stake: her children, her job, and, most of all, her reputation. She must appear to be in control. Most probably, the people around her are acutely aware of these everyday realities, while the daily, hidden drudgery of her life 'under the influence' affects them to varying degrees. With a deceptive public face she masks a private, painful face known only to herself and perhaps these few significant others.

Breaking out of this ring of deception takes courage and self-understanding. One needs to find the courage to believe that this promise of the good life' is able to come from oneself, not one's bottle. Also, self-understanding fosters a sense of loyalty or being true to oneself. It helps to expose self-betrayal. One expert[22] has suggested that a woman needs to 'reverse' the feelings that made her drink and start having good feelings about herself. Women will stop betraying themselves only if they experience loyalty more from themselves than from a bottle of alcohol.

WOMEN'S COMPOUNDED PROBLEMS

Racism, classism, ageism, heterosexism and every other social pattern of inequality that erodes women's power, their courage, their integrity and their self-esteem contribute to the complexities of their relationship to alcohol. Here, I suggest that women drinkers' problems become compounded by prejudices about these social inequalities. As we have seen, negative drinking contradicts society's ideals of feminine behaviour. In many instances, women who experience negative drinking unknowingly bring into their lives a whole series of physical, emotional and relational problems. Their unique position in society – with all of the forced stereotypes, roles and expectations about women who overdrink – is not the only factor that affects their relationships.

For example, if a woman is poor or working-class, she may appear to be less worthy of help, compassion or protection than an overdrinking woman who has more material assets or more access to economic and political resources. Unfortunately, this attitude, although at times camouflaged, runs very deep in our society.

A woman of colour may experience a different hidden message. Regardless of her specific ethnic background, she may experience either blatant or invisible racism. Whether obtrusive or hidden, racism confronting a woman who overdrinks has the potential to make her life even more painful than it is. The experience of racism, in any form, compounds her problems. One woman of colour who had experienced negative drinking for two years said:

> I really hate now the charming pictures of black women in alcohol ads. All of that glamour. That's not it . . . Booze is different in our culture . . . These pictures, these ads are white people's . . . Just try being a drunk black woman in public . . . you'll see what I mean.

Another inequality, the issue of age, is rarely considered as a compounding problem in our drinking culture. Never-theless, hidden ageism exists, and its effects are most probably felt more often by women than men drinkers. One woman clarifies this point:

> I have been thinking about women and drinking. You know there is also an age thing. Take a group of, say, 23-

year-olds. Your average 23-year-old in Europe will be out disco-ing and drinking and going to the pub, bar, whatever . . . Females and males will be drinking the same amounts. But, look at drinkers who are older – say in their fifties. If a woman in her fifties is drinking as much as a man in his fifties then she is viewed as a bad woman. But for some reason a woman in her twenties who is drinking the same amount as a man in his twenties is one of the gang. It is just accepted, this age discrimination.

Besides the above patterns of social inequality, overdrinking women who are lesbian may experience further discrimination, based on their sexual orientation. As mentioned previously, alcohol has become an acceptable socialising substance in parts of the lesbian sub-culture, while drinking to the point of being mildly intoxicated or even drunk is often considered perfectly acceptable at specific social events. In talking with lesbians, one finds that many if not most 'out' lesbians[23] prefer to drink in the company of other lesbians or gay men. Simply, many lesbians want to socialise in well-defined spaces (eg bars, clubs, discos, etc) frequented solely by lesbians and/or gay men. This enables them to socialise freely without the fear of being discriminated against because of their sexual orientation. While there are various ways of drinking in the lesbian sub-culture, a lesbian who experiences negative drinking may find it safer, both physically and psychologically, to overdrink within the narrow confines of the well-defined spaces of the lesbian sub-culture. While her overdrinking may not be fully understood by those around her, she avoids the sorts of recrimination, verbal abuse and physical attack that could result from her being drunk in public and/or in mainly heterosexual bars, pubs or drinking places. While members of the lesbian sub-culture may not condone continuous overdrinking, they look more sympathetically at lesbian overdrinkers than does the average male or female heterosexual drinking in public bars.

One lesbian recalls an intense experience she had in the lesbian drinking culture in a large English city:

> We used to meet for almost two years in the top of this pub . . . We had a large room for dancing on Friday and Saturday nights. It was the first time I ever had lager with Scotch chasers. Sometimes we had to wait for the upstairs room to open so we would wait downstairs. There were mostly men there and it was hard to get a drink downstairs. I always knew there would be comments. If any lesbian came in drunk, it was a problem. This was because in order to get upstairs we had to get in first downstairs. If a lesbian would come in drunk, we would whisk her upstairs. Once it got nasty and there was some violence. A lesbian was beaten up by a gang of young boys. That's when the owner decided to ban us from the pub.

SPECIAL GROUPS OF WOMEN

When we consider the complexities of women's use of alcohol, there are groups of women who may need to be studied further. In the following discussion we look briefly at women who work in high 'alcohol risk' jobs such as sex workers, bartenders, cocktail waitresses and flight attendants, as well as at housewives and nuns, who have a particularly high investment in keeping their overdrinking hidden.

Let us focus first on women in high 'alcohol risk' jobs. They can be seen as being in high 'alcohol risk' jobs because their work exposes them to alcohol in a risky way.[24] They tend to work in environments where alcohol flows more freely than usual. For example, some women who work in the sex industry may find that an important part of their work is not only to provide sexual services to predominantly male clients but also to socialise with them in an atmosphere where drinking, and at times overdrinking, is encouraged.

Women bartenders and cocktail waitresses may find that their work involves accepting alcoholic drinks from customers who reward them for their service. Also, flight attendants work in an atmosphere in which alcoholic beverages are more often than not encouraged as a way of helping customers cope with the fear of flying, general claustrophobia, boredom or relaxation. This, combined with the stress of the work and difficult schedules, can make the job a high 'alcohol risk'. One woman who was a flight attendant discussed her experience and described herself as one of the 'lucky ones' who had a 'close call' with alcohol, which nearly cost her job:

> I was one of the lucky ones. I didn't lose my job because I had a drink problem, but some did. My problem started very slowly and it really began when I started the long-haul journeys. We were kept quite busy for nearly the whole flight. It was stressful work and I started drinking as a way of getting to sleep after we landed – I felt it calmed me . . . I started to drink secretly on the job. I did not drink heavily but enough that it showed. I was lucky because my supervisor suggested that I become involved in the Employee Assistance Programme. It was a new programme that had been set up for those of us who had drink problems. So, I began alcohol counselling and it really helped me to look at my drinking and see why I was drinking so much. I was transferred to shorter flights after that. Now my drinking is under control and I only drink on weekends – never while I am working – but it was a close call.

Overdrinking interferes with the caring or servicing role that most, if not all, women are expected to be involved in to some extent. Some women may try to hide their overdrinking and avoid being stigmatised as 'bad carers'. Whether or not attempts are made to hide their overdrinking, women whose lives are more isolated than others may find their alcohol problems remain very hidden. In this context let us look at two other groups of women: housewives and nuns. Let us focus first on housewives.

When discussing the issue of alcohol and women's relationships earlier in this chapter, we saw that secret drinking involved women in a whole series of emotions (eg shame, guilt, denial and fear) that took time to become visible. We also saw that some of these secret drinkers were housewives. Secrecy is absolutely crucial for these women because it allows them to maintain their housewife roles and the facade that they are coping well with their daily duties. One woman gave the example of a friend who was a housewife and a secret drinker:

> There is the example of [name] – a housewife and mother of four children. She was doing all the things she was supposed to do. She took the children to school; she got them to their sports club; she chauffeured them around and she worked for her husband who was a doctor. All the time, she was topping up on alcohol in private.

This particular housewife appeared to function well, while her negative drinking was hidden. But the time eventually came when her overdrinking interfered with her caring duties, and she needed help. But to ask for help meant that she would be stigmatised and seen as an irresponsible, bad mother. As we already know, asking for help is often difficult for any woman, but for the overdrinking housewife, asking for help may expose her very well-kept secret. It can be a devastating experience in which she feels a total failure.

Another group of women who have a high investment in keeping their overdrinking secret is nuns. Generally their personal problems remain hidden from society because they live quite isolated lives. Also, there is much mystery associated with convent life. If a nun develops an alcohol problem, it is seen as quite unusual. But nuns do develop alcohol problems. It is easier now than in the past for a variety of reasons: the general openness of contemporary religious life; the frequent if not daily partaking of alcohol (ie wine at Mass) and the possibility of maintaining extreme secrecy if one wants to overdrink.

One woman I spoke to, an ex-nun, knew two nuns who had an alcohol problem and enjoyed drinking secretly in their bedrooms. Because this ex-nun saw neither of these two nuns drunk, she was unable to ascertain their level of dependence upon alcohol. However, she recalled that one nun was notorious for falling down and hurting herself. She also remembered that both nuns were in their late sixties, had been retired from teaching for a few years and, therefore, had quite a lot of free time which they used for drinking:

> It was quite common for Sister [name] and Sister [name] to drink in secret during what was called their private time. They usually did this after doing the daily housework. Even though they were retired, they would help the other nuns with their chores . . . Both Sisters had refrigerators in their private bedrooms. I remember that when they showed me the contents of their refrigerators, they kept alcohol in them. I also remember that the alcohol was spirits, either whisky or gin. I thought at the time that it was a little odd, but I never gave it too much thought. I do not know how much they were drinking in private or if they drank with each other. It was only when

I started to hear of [one of the Sister's name]'s falls that I made the connection between drinking and those falls. I knew then it was the effects of the alcohol.

This ex-nun said that alcohol was kept in the convent for specific reasons – it was used as a sleeping remedy, for example, and 'altar wine' was allowed during daily Mass. Otherwise, drinking was prohibited and a general atmosphere of temperance prevailed. That is why the two Sisters felt they needed to keep their drinking a secret.

This chapter has outlined and discussed the types of multiple problems that women involved in negative drinking experience on the bodily, emotional and relational levels. It has also shown how these problems are often compounded by different patterns of inequality, such as racism, classism, ageism and heterosexism, existing in society.

I suggest that women, whether they are non-drinkers, moderate drinkers or overdrinkers, must learn to recognise these multiple problems so as to help develop a collective sense of concern. In turn, this concern allows women drinkers, particularly those involved in negative drinking, to begin to focus on hope rather than despair. On the other hand, all those concerned with the women and alcohol issue may begin to appreciate and to understand more fully that women's drinking can be seen through women-sensitive eyes.

Notes

1. In describing the pervasiveness of the problems faced by women dependent upon alcohol or other drugs, S. Murphy and M. Rosenbaum speak of 'polyproblems'. See their 'Editors'

Introduction', *Journal of Psychoactive Drugs* 19, 2 (1987): 125–28. I have used this term in my previous work with special reference to alcohol. See Elizabeth Ettorre, *Women and Substance Use* (London: Macmillan and New Brunswick NJ: Rutgers University Press, 1992), Chapter Two, 'Women and alcohol' pp 32–51.

2. Marilyn Mason uses this concept, internalised shame, to demonstrate how shame, born in relationship to others, becomes internalised in women alcoholics' lives. See her 'Women and Shame: Kin and Culture' in Claudia Bepko, ed, *Feminism and Addiction* (New York, London and Sydney: The Haworth Press, 1991).

3. One of the first pieces of writing that showed these differences quite clearly was Brigid McConville's *Women Under the Influence: Alcohol and its Impact* (New York: Shocken Books, 1983).

4. The word 'gendered' is used here to mean that society's view of what is acceptable for men who drink and women who drink varies. This view is based on social expectations of what is seen as being appropriate for the sexes .

5. Experts in the alcohol field talk about alcohol as being both physically and psychologically addictive. A classic discussion in this area is included in The Royal College of Psychiatrists, *Alcohol and Alcoholism: Report of a Special Commission* (London: Tavistock, 1979).

6. See R Norton, T Dwyer and S Macmahon, 'Alcohol Consumption and the Risk of Alcohol-Related Cirrhosis in Women', *British Medical Journal* 295 (1987): 80–82.

7. CG Harper, NA Smith and JJ Kril, 'The Effects of Alcohol on the Human Brain: a Neuropathological Study', *Alcohol* 25 (1990): 445–48.

8. See Rosemary Kent, *Say When!: Everything a Woman Needs to Know about Alcohol and Drinking Problems* (London: Sheldon Press, 1990), especially Chapter Five, 'How much is too much?', pp 34–49, for an interesting discussion on this issue.

9. I have already explained in the introduction my dislike of the term 'alcoholic'. I should add here that I am critical of the term 'addict'. This is because I have heard others use this word to hurt people, both men and women. So for me it has a negative meaning. However, 'addict' can be used positively, as it is very often by members of Narcotics Anonymous (NA). Throughout this book I use 'addict' only for descriptive purposes.

10. This tends to be a taboo area of discussion in the alcohol field. One

is hard pressed to find any evidence of this. My view comes from observations of women both in alcohol and drug treatment settings and comparisons of their physical conditions. In a related context, Sarah Hafner, *Nice Girls Don't Drink: Stories of Recovery* (New York: Bergin and Garvey, 1992), describes the lives of women who have recovered from alcohol abuse. Mary's story (pp 64–75) is an eye-opening one of someone who abused both alcohol and illegal drugs (speed, mescaline and pills). In her case, alcohol appeared to have a worse effect on her body than the illegal drugs she consumed .

11. Katherine van Wormer, *Alcoholism Treatment: A Social Work Perspective* (Chicago: Nelson Hall Publishers, 1995), p 103.

12. Sarah Hafner, *Nice Girls Don' t Drink*, p 209.

13. See, for example, David Berenson, 'Powerlessness-liberating or Enslaving? Responding to the Feminist Critique of the Twelve Steps', in Claudia Bepko, ed, *Feminism and Addiction*.

14. Sheila Ernst and Lucy Goodison, attempting to recognise the historical dimensions of women's subordination, have noted that women have been brought up to be submissive to and supportive of others. They also note that caring, loving, emotional and practical support are expected from women and that women are expected to be the carriers of emotions. See Sheila Ernst and Lucy Goodison, *In Our Own Hands: A Book of Self-Help Therapy* (London: The Women's Press, 1981), pp 1–10.

15. See, for example, Jean Kirkpatrick, *Turnabout: New Help for the Woman Alcoholic* (Seattle: Madrona Publishers, 1986), for interesting insights in this area.

16. See Sandra Lee Bartsky, *Femininity and Domination* (New York and London: Routledge, 1990), specifically Chapter Six, 'Shame and gender', pp 83–98, where she demonstrates how shame is related to gender.

17. Sandra Lee Bartsky, *Femininity and Domination*.

18. See Patricia Pasick and Christine White, 'Challenging General Patton: A Feminist Stance in Substance Abuse Treatment and Training' in Claudia Bepko, ed, *Feminism and Addiction*. Here 'active denial' suggests an active resistance rather than total blocking of emotions.

19. I refer to an excellent article by Dusty Miller, 'Are We Keeping up with Oprah?: A Treatment and Training Model for Addictions and Interpersonal Violence', in Claudia Bepko, ed, *Feminism and Addiction*. Here, Miller emphasises the need to keep an open mind in

relation to women who may be the recipients and givers of violence as well as having been traumatised at some time in their lives. Simply, moralising about these women is harmful to the healing or therapeutic process.

20. This is perhaps one of the reasons why AA is strictly anonymous. It is a way of protecting members from public shame.

21. JL Forth Finegan, 'Sugar and Spice and Everything Nice: Gender Socialization and Women's Addiction – A Literature Review' in Claudia Bepko, ed, *Feminism and Addiction,* pp 28–29.

22. See Sarah Hafner, *Nice Girls Don't Drink,* p 160, where Jean Kirkpatrick talks about this type of change in her story of recovery.

23. Here I use the term 'out' in the traditional sense – to refer to those lesbians who have in some way declared publicly that they are lesbians.

24. In a classic article, Shirley Otto provides an overview of studies on female habitual drunken offenders. The literature exposes some links between prostitution and drunkenness. See Otto, 'Single Homeless Women and Alcohol', in Camberwell Council on Alcoholism, *Women and Alcohol* (London and New York: Tavistock, 1980).

CHAPTER 3

Multiple images and social hypocrisy

For too long, women's health has been governed by persons other than themselves . . . Women for Sobriety challenges women to learn their strengths and values, to become aware that they are competent women, that sobriety depends upon the discovery and maintenance of strong feelings of self-worth which, ultimately, will lead to strong self-esteem . . . We who are alcoholics used alcohol to cope with the problems and stresses of life. When we find we must live without alcohol, we must then learn other ways to cope with those problems. We must identify our strengths to do this, and develop these strengths to their utmost. For women, this presents special problems because so few have enough self-confidence or sense of themselves as competent human beings . . . People still begin drinking for the same reasons. Many men drink to feel powerful, to feel masterful, to feel in charge; women seem to drink from feelings of inadequacy, of loneliness, frustration and depression.[1]

These words were spoken by Jean Kirkpatrick, who in the late 1970s in the USA established Women for Sobriety because she believed that AA did not meet the needs of everyone, especially women. Her view is that we need to take charge of our own problems with alcohol and see that our needs differ significantly from those of male alcoholics. Furthermore, she believed that our needs as women have been consistently ignored in general ideas on alcoholism. For example, important issues such as domestic stress; violence against women; sexual abuse; gender role conflict; recreational drug use and a recognition of women's multiple problems as well as the power of multiple negative images have remained hidden, if not completely overlooked in the alcohol field.

Those who use traditional approaches in alcohol studies examine alcohol predominantly from a male point of view. Thus, women are marginalised and viewed purely within a domestic setting – as an appendage to men within the family.[2] Furthermore, when examining the relationship between male alcoholics and their female partners, many experts see wives as acting out destructive and/or masochistic behaviour. Max Glatt provides an overview of how the wives of alcoholics are portrayed in the literature of alcohol studies and mentions the following prevalent images: 'Suffering Susan', 'Controlling Catherine', 'Wavering Winifred' and 'Punitive Polly' – images that suggest that wives are often blamed for their husbands' alcoholism.[3] So the particular problems women alcoholics face are not dealt with, while the problems of male alcoholics are often blamed, in some way, on their wives. Since the female alcoholic is considered much more dangerous than the male alcoholic (see pp 14–16), it seems that women cannot win. Whether as alcoholics or as wives of alcoholics, women are seen to be more destructive than men.

A DOUBLE STANDARD OR SOCIAL HYPOCRISY?

If alcohol is involved in any social situation where men and women are involved, you are immediately dealing with double standards. This is my own experience because for many years I was involved with a man who was an alcoholic too.

The above words were spoken by a woman who had experienced negative drinking for 15 years. Over the years, she learned why she needed to drink so much. She was also familiar with the problems that followed on from overdrinking. She joined AA. However, from her viewpoint as a woman, she was critical of how she had been judged, feeling that she had been treated more severely in comparison to the man she was involved with. Her words suggest that there are different sets of moral judgements used to define men's and women's use of alcohol. More often than not these judgements reveal a clear, social bias in favour of men.

People active in the alcohol field have continually discussed this as the double standard,[4] referring to the use of two sets of rules for alcohol use in society: one for men and the other for women. Within this view, women who overdrink are seen to deny well-defined female images or stereotypes[5] and to reject the norms (ie unwritten rules) for an average woman, while a man who overdrinks is viewed as being 'one of the boys'.

Concerning this latter view, the woman quoted above also talked about how alcohol establishes maleness or masculinity. She gives an example of 'her man', an Irishman, who needed to prove himself through alcohol:

He was the son of an Irish cop in [city name]. He was the first generation of his family to ever go near to a high school. His family did not have any education. So he prided himself on knowing how to dress. He was a salesman and he had an education. He was charm personified but he was a lush – just like his old man. So we would get absolutely pissed together. I picked him up in a bar . . . But I know he used to think conventionally that if an Irishman can't drink he is a wimp as a man . . . handling your liquor is a really manly, macho kind of thing. Never mind that you get pissed all the time.

This woman recalled that alcohol was what bound them together, and their bond was in reality an 'alcoholic bond'. She says quite frankly:

. . . Although we were lovers, we had a sick alcoholic relationship, an alcoholic bond. He was an Irish lush. But, as a woman, I was seen as more of a disgrace than him when I started to drink uncontrollably. When we broke up, I left [city name] and came back home.

So a drinking man and a drinking woman are treated differently. This double standard runs very deep. As one woman said:

It is OK for a man to drink more than a woman – to be drunk. It has always been like that for me. I knew it. I cannot explain how that feeling came about because I do not remember my parents or anybody else consciously talking about it. I just know I knew it.

There is more to this double standard than meets the eye. Both unwritten and written laws legislating the ways that men and women are expected to behave in society are gendered; ie if we look at any number of social images of bad, evil and immoral individuals, we find these images differ according to whether we are focusing on men or women. When a woman acts in a way that puts her outside of the boundaries of acceptable feminine behaviour, she is seen as unfeminine, anti-social or deviant. Of course, if a man acts in a comparable way, stepping outside of the boundaries of masculinity, he is viewed similarly according to male standards. However, I would argue that the spaces for acting out acceptable masculine behaviour are numerous compared to the spaces for acceptable feminine behaviour. Women's behaviour is more bounded by social sanctions and norms and thus, women tend to be judged more harshly than men.

One woman I spoke to felt quite strongly that women are simply not allowed to lose control and be drunk in society. She herself finds it difficult to cope with a drunken woman, in spite of having experienced negative drinking. She expressed her judgemental attitudes quite openly:

> If a woman is drunk, it is very obvious how she will be treated and judged. People make many more moral judgements about drunken women than drunken men. I do it. I cannot help it. That is the way it is. It is just not allowed for women – any woman – to be drunk.

Clearly, harsh moral judgements can be made about any drunken displays in public. But, in comparison to men, women experience harsher moral judgements when they are involved in drunken displays.

One woman talked about the anger that women's public drunkenness can arouse:

> I think people are slightly disgusted or even angry when a woman is drunk. A woman's drunkenness causes anger in others.

If women do become drunk in public, this 'out of control' behaviour is viewed as innapropriate and best contained within the private spaces of the home. One woman emphasised this quite explicitly when she said:

> If you start to see a woman getting drunk and being loud and acting obnoxious and spilling her drinks all over the

place or whatever, this seems to create a negative feeling in those around her. The message is, 'Doesn't she know she is making a fool of herself and she should go home?'

Another woman echoed this point when she said:

When a woman is drunk, I mean really drunk, I usually see it as being a case of 'Someone should take her home' or 'It is time for you to go home now, dear – you're making a fool of yourself'.

The above woman spoke about how sad she felt when she observed drunken women in public. She felt sad because she believed that no one was ever interested in why a particular woman needed to get drunk. She believed that people only got embarrassed or angry, did not show concern or compassion, and tended to respond in superficial ways. In her view, most people uphold traditional social conventions: a woman's drunken behaviour is best contained within the home. People don't ask why the woman is drunk or try to look beyond the drunken behaviour, and this was somewhat problematic for her:

No one has ever really asked these women, 'Why are you drinking so much?' Of course, every now and again you think to yourself, 'I wonder why she is drinking too much?' You may think, 'Maybe she has a problem' or 'Does she have a problem?' But I have never heard it said out loud, 'Why is she drinking too much?' What people say tends to be on the surface – for that occasion. They say, 'You are drunk'; 'Go home'; 'You are making a fool of yourself' and so on. It is this kind of attitude. It is never, 'You are drunk and you are making a fool of yourself and why are you doing this?' Why never comes into it.

The above accounts suggest that 'sending a woman home'

appears to remove her from humiliation and social shame, but also from public visibility. They also suggest that 'sending a woman home' is returning her to her rightful place, the private arena, the home, domestic life in which control and compliance can, perhaps, be re-established. While she may be removed from public view, she is not removed from the private gaze of her partner or husband and family, if she has one. At the very least, 'sending a woman home' places her more directly under the scrutiny of her family's watchful eyes, if she overdrinks.

We are beginning to see here that the way we react to women's overdrinking reflects our social attitudes to women. Women should not be out of control; they should not make a display of themselves in public; if a woman is not behaving well, she must be sent back to her family, to whom she is responsible.

On the other hand, when women overdrink and lose control of themselves in private, they may no longer be able to be controlled by another. Their feminine obedience or female conformity may be called into question. Also, they may be unable to care for those around them when they overdrink. Since women more often than men are responsible for caring for others, this can be considered a very serious matter. The stress, anxieties, difficulties and emotions women may have experienced prior to their negative drinking are rarely foregrounded; rather, these women appear as failures in their moral duty to maintain their feminine and maternal responsibilities.

It is still the case that women more than men are supposed to hold the moral high ground. However old fashioned it may seem, women more than men are assumed to be symbols of moral purity. In this way, women are not only the emotional carers, carriers and copers, but also the custodians, champions, caretakers and guardians of morals within society. If a woman falls from social grace she falls harder and further than a man. Her unfeminine, anti-social or deviant behaviour signals in some way moral decay.[6] In the area of moral judgements, men, therefore, tend to have much more 'moral leeway' than women because the boundaries separating acceptable public and private conduct are much wider for men than for women.

For example, when a man is a rapist, thief, bank robber, white-collar criminal, mugger, drug addict, pimp, etc, he may find that activities linked to these unacceptable roles establish rather than threaten his masculinity. If a woman is involved in similar activities, she is viewed as not only less good (ie more immoral) than her male equal but also as a failure as a mother, wife, carer, human.

As the standard-bearers of morals, women are supposed to focus on nurturing and caring for others, partly if not mainly in the privacy of the home. Regardless of whether or not women have paid work outside the home, women more than men have the responsibility to take care of the private world of the household, the children and the family. On the other hand, men are the protectors and standard-bearers of subsistence, maintaining the visible, social order, the public area. This has particular effects on how society views women's drinking in comparison to men's because, although society often appears not to value the private sphere as much as the public sphere – going out to work is often regarded as more important than staying at home with the children and the housework – in fact, looking after the home and family carries powerful social and moral significance. For example, the family is viewed as the basic emotional and economic unit in society, and an overdrinking wife and mother unable to cope with her domestic duties can be considered a threat to that.

On a more personal level, a man or woman may lose a

job, a good reputation, friends, etc, but more often than not, if the private area of the home/family is jeopardised in any way, this threat is perceived as a danger to the equilibrium of society.

So what the above tells us is that wherever women drink, either in public or private, they are seen to have lost control. Women more than men are not allowed to lose control. If they do, they will suffer a much more powerful reaction against them.

This is social hypocrisy and it is a hypocrisy that needs to be observed when we discuss women's relationship to alcohol. This social hypocrisy distorts the real picture of women who drink and ensures that overdrinking women carry a much bigger burden than their male counterparts.

MULTIPLE IMAGES

Alongside a deep social hypocrisy comes the creation of over-simplified images of women who drink, whether negatively or positively. What is behind the creation of images of women's negative drinking? In my view, the images attached to overdrinking women are so numerous that one can only speak of 'multiple images'. For example, there is the drunken whore, the loose woman, the female lush, the weak woman, the evil woman, the liberated woman, the bad mother, the boisterous woman, the lusty woman, the out-of-control woman, and so on.

That these images have been created shows us how overdrinking women are pigeonholed into representations of disgraceful women. Their disgrace or stigma is based on moral judgements and ideas about acceptable drinking conduct as well as acceptable women. Similar to the issue of multiple problems, discussed in the previous chapter, the issue of multiple images creates difficulties for many women. In pinpointing these multiple images, we need to go below the surface of what is immediately visible in the lives of overdrinking women. Multiple images tend to be extremely deep within society, and therefore they are difficult to uncover.

But who are these drunken whores, these female lushes, these bad mothers, these loose, weak, evil, liberated, boisterous, lusty, out-of-control, wild, flirtatious, desperate, lost, lonely, pathetic, and living-in-an-empty-nest women? Simply, they are the women who become the targets of extreme social disapproval by the very fact that they overdrink. They are the women whose images of themselves tend to become distorted because these images are imposed upon them by others who hold rigid judgements. Whether or not these negative images may have some basis in real life is not the issue. For example, some women may actually feel more psychologically, sexually or socially free – even wild – after they consume an inordinate amount of alcohol. This is not the point. The main point is that these images stigmatise the women who are targeted. Additionally, targeting these women is all about making them feel that in order to be morally upstanding women, they need to be not only better but also more in control of their liquor intake than men.

One woman describes her impression that women are expected to be examples of purity and social control when alcohol is around. In her mind, these issues are closely linked:

> Women are supposed to be like the Virgin Mary. They are not supposed to get into trouble. They are not supposed to behave that way – to lose control and get drunk. So if a woman behaves that way, it is frowned on. That is how she is looked upon. A drinking man – you would simply

pass by. It's not the same for him. But a woman, say a woman who is visibly drunk, it goes against the idea that women do not get drunk in public.

These words suggest that overdrinking women violate many if not all the cherished ideals of what it means to be a woman, feminine and female in contemporary society. Social decorum, etiquette, compliance, submission, purity, and a graceful social demeanour are all required for women to be seen as virtuous and upstanding. These features appear to have gone out of the window the moment a woman becomes drunk. But regardless of whether or not women drink, we all share the same social commandments to be virtuous and above reproach as well as be the guardians of moral and social values. These social commandments have been preserved over the ages because men more than women have had the power to legitimate morality and legislate social standards and, in turn, to define acceptability for women. Women who overdrink offer a special threat to these traditional female roles. They are seen as having deserted respectability in most if not every area of their lives.

These sorts of ideas are ingrained in many women from a very early age. Clear messages are received, for example, from the books we read or the movies we see. However, while these messages may appear to be plain or uncomplicated, they instill in many women distorted images of their relationship to alcohol.

In this context, it is interesting to refer to the comments of one woman who recalled her experience of reading novels in her youth. She remembered that most authors inevitably made a distinction between the woman who drank moderately and the woman who was a drunk. She also suggested that how women characters drank was linked up with the presence or absence of female virtue. She says:

I was just recalling reading books where the female characters in the novels were always above drunkenness and bad conduct – that is to say that they didn't drink too much. Maybe they would take a drink or two and that was it. But, if there was drunkenness in novels, it was always the bad girl from down the road or the other side of the tracks. She was the one who slept around . . . She was not the heroine. We tend to think, 'What heroine would do that?'

Another powerful medium that has shaped the distorted images of women who overdrink has been film. Here, the stigmas are very clear and women are often portrayed as being lonesome, sad, lacking self-confidence, destructive and dependent. An excellent article called 'Women, Alcohol and the Screen' demonstrates this.[7]

In discussing popular images that are presented as the 'truth', we begin to see that for women these multiple images can magnify as well as multiply the painful effects of negative drinking. In my experience of talking with women about the pain of their negative drinking, I have found that powerful disapproving images will inevitably block the healing process. For example, if a woman wants to reduce or stop her overdrinking, these images may not only increase her guilt and shame, but also heighten her hurt. While she needs to deal with these overwhelming images, she also needs to heal herself. If she is unable to deal with these multiple images because of the feelings they arouse, she will soon discover that a potentially rich, healing process becomes blocked. Clearly, because a double standard exists, women experience these images as stigmas; the effect is more distressing, more lasting and indeed more destructive than for men.

BLOCKING THE HEALING PROCESS

I suggested in the above discussion that pejorative images place a stigma on women who are targeted and that these multiple images serve to devalue women's experiences and, in turn, block a healing process. Women who overdrink may actually feel that they have been bad mothers, loose, weak, evil, liberated, boisterous, lusty, out of control, wild, flirtatious, desperate, lost, lonely, pathetic, and so on. Perhaps, on some level, they have been any one or more of these kinds of women. Simply, they are able to identify with one or more of these images and view their own lives in a similar fashion. My main point here is that if these multiple images or labels actually stick, it can be very difficult for any woman not only to remove them but also to move beyond them to more positive images of herself. Most important, it becomes impossible for her to really value herself when these labels are glued on to her by society.

Regardless of whether or not these images are based on reality, the actual everyday lives of women who overdrink need to be re-framed by themselves as well as by society. Creating multiple negative images is all about devaluing women. But many if not most women have been taught to devalue themselves in some way. For example, our bodies, our feelings, our emotions, our ethics, our work, our caring, etc, are often seen as not good enough in relation to men and sometimes each other.

One woman spoke about how most women have not been allowed to show themselves as strong, powerful or aggressive. In her view, women are only valued for being less good or weaker both physically and psychologically than men. This makes it doubly difficult for women who experience negative drinking to value themselves. She believed that in order for women to overcome such a huge problem, women need to learn a way of valuing themselves. For her, if women could learn this, they could be better able to heal themselves. She says:

> . . . I think this whole women and alcohol issue is very painful. I think that the way women have been brought up is not to value themselves – not to have this great powerful ego or person: you know, the stiff upper lip, the 'I have got to show myself to be strong and defended'. Men have this sense. We women have not been valued in that way . . . The subtle thing is (and this is difficult to explain) that we need to re-frame women who are seen as victims. We need to take a new look at their devaluing, their experiences and so on. We need to say that out of this devaluing can be born something of value. Yes, there is much suffering. I say this not as a way of devaluing women. It means that in this pile of muck something good can come of it for women.

To make something good come out of 'this pile of muck' is to learn the art, the craft or the skill of healing. Women learn this skill in the face of unacceptable images which they confront and which devalue their lives as overdrinking women. Learning to heal is learning to feel good enough. In addition, to learn healing is to learn how to overturn these devaluing images.

RECOGNISING DEVALUING AND NEGATIVE IMAGES

Before looking at how to overturn negative images, we need to recognise the hidden realities which often exist behind these images. Here, I will digress slightly to look at a very powerful negative image that links alcohol with women's sexuality, as well as other popular images of drinking women.

A very convincing image attached to women who overdrink is that they are sexually promiscuous. Simply, female *alcohol* intemperance is seen to be equal to female *sexual* intemperance. In fact, links are sometimes made between women's overdrinking and prostitution. Thus we have the labels the 'drunken whore' or 'drunken slut'. On the one hand, a drunken woman does not need to be a prostitute to have a promiscuous image. She is viewed already as sexually promiscuous by the very fact that she is a drunk. On the other hand, a prostitute who may also be a 'drunk' is viewed as doubly promiscuous because she overdrinks as well as works in the sex industry.

While it may be hard for some women to challenge these images and break this link between being drunk and being seen as oversexed, it is possible at least to understand the truth in the link between consuming alcohol and feeling uninhibited, whether sexually, emotionally, psychologically or socially. Remember alcohol is a drug. It has physical effects and it can and does release some of our hidden feelings and emotions. For women, their first step in breaking the link between alcohol and sex is to recognise that this link exists. The next step is to understand that, for any person, a woman or a man, experiencing a release of inhibitions does not automatically mean that this release is of a sexual nature. There are many ways to be uninhibited, just as there are many ways to drink alcohol. To feel uninhibited can be a very basic human feeling. To be uninhibited may feel like freedom.

One woman I spoke with had been a negative drinker for four years. Now she speaks about the 'pleasant feelings' that alcohol creates in 'her body and mind'. She uses alcohol in a controlled way and calls herself a 'moderate drinker'. If she gets intoxicated, it is at most once a year – either on Christmas or New Year's Eve. On the whole, alcohol makes her feel free and uninhibited. She says she needs some kind of release and alcohol is her drug. She feels that this kind of release is important to her because she has a 'very stressful job' as a community worker. She is dealing continually with other people's problems. She says:

> In the past when I was drinking a lot, I was too wild at parties – I was not coping. I drank alcohol because I could not cope with my feelings or because I wanted to calm myself or get what I wanted – like to have sex with someone to avoid loneliness. I drank a lot then and my drinking was mixed with having sex . . . Now I feel free when I drink. If I can have a drink in the afternoon, it means that I am free to take it. That is why when I am on holiday, the first thing I do regardless of the time of the day is to have a drink. This is because alcohol symbolises freedom to me. Now I am free from all of my duties that are on my mind when I work.

This woman's story shows an interesting lesson that she learned. While she was able to break the link between alcohol and sex in her own life, she came to understand her need to feel free, released or uninhibited. These feelings are not of a sexual nature as they may have appeared to be in her past life. In contrast to her earlier experiences, she drinks for pleasure and to feel free. While drinking means she will feel uninhibited, it no longer means acting out her sexual inhibitions. While she may obviously have sexual feelings during as well as outside of times of drinking, she does not automatically jump into bed with anyone around her.

Besides 'the drunken whore' or 'the slut' images, other popular images can include the 'bad mother'; 'irresponsible wife'; 'evil woman'; 'loose woman'; 'suburban housewife'; 'menopausal woman'; 'liberated young college girl' and 'harassed woman executive'. Let us study these briefly. A woman who experiences negative drinking can be seen to be in private a 'bad mother', uncaring for her children, or an 'irresponsible wife', not considering the needs of her partner or husband. In public, she is viewed as unforgivably out of control of her domestic and/or work situation, or maybe as an 'evil' or 'loose' woman who cannot be trusted.

Images such as 'the suburban housewife' who is bored and frustrated or 'the menopausal woman', living 'in an empty nest' where she feels abandoned by her working husband and her adult children, can be based on the real experiences of some women who overdrink. Added to this list of images are 'the liberated young college girl' and 'the harassed woman executive', images suggesting that women may be adapting a more masculine than feminine drinking conduct. However, whether or not contemporary women have greater social freedom, including the freedom to drink, than women in the past does not suggest that the stigma attached to women's drinking has disappeared. We should aim to abolish altogether negative images of women's drinking rather than to slap these labels on women or create new images. This means that we need to nurture a women-sensitive awareness of the links between women and alcohol. While times have changed, social attitudes towards overdrinking woman have been continually about creating shameful images, that, unfortunately, stick.

OVERTURNING DEVALUING AND NEGATIVE IMAGES

In order to overturn negative images, we first need to understand them. Why do they exist? Is there some truth to them? How can we change them and overturn them? If we do not need them, what sorts of images can we use in their place? What images can be useful for healing?

Here we have 'the pathetic woman' character.[8] She is a white, divorced, employed woman in her late fifties who drinks daily. She is often under the influence of alcohol at her workplace. On the surface she is a very kind woman but she is easily bullied and dominated. For her, drinking alcohol is an emotional crutch, propping her up and helping her to deal with criticism and sometimes verbal abuse from others. Her conduct brings out pity from others, but she actually feels pity towards herself. She lives the life of a pathetic woman. Her life is a misery. For her, a less hurtful image of herself could be a 'woman in pain', pain that has increased over the years through her own timidity and lack of social skills. Although a public display of pain in our society is not very valued, women more than men are allowed to show, if not express publicly, their pain. But for any man or woman this is a highly sensitive area.

The main point here is that showing pain, tenderness or vulnerability for this woman can be all about showing her strength. This is because vulnerability is not a sign of weakness but a sign of strength. In this light, being seen as vulnerable for this woman can be more highly valued than being seen as pathetic. A recognition of vulnerability by herself and those around her allows for empathy rather than pity to be awakened in others.

For our next image, we have the 'boisterous, aggressive lush'. She is a 25-year-old, white, employed and divorced woman. She is quite dependent upon alcohol although she is unable to admit it. On every social occasion, she always wants to go to the pub. For her, every social occasion is an occasion to drink. She consistently gets drunk and is quite aggressive and argumentative. She quarrels with those around her. Her conduct brings out anger and contempt from others, but she actually feels anger and contempt towards herself. She lives the life of a loud-mouthed woman.

Her life is full of aggression. For her, a less hurtful image of herself could be 'an assertive woman', a woman who begins to focus on what she wants — a difficult area in any woman's life. Accepting this image means that others will begin to see her energy, an energy that is vibrant and full of wanting. Rather than awakening contempt and anger, her energy is focused. In searching for what she really wants, she allows herself to move from a desperate seeking of others' attention to a lively, difficult and challenging kind of seeking. Overturning this image can mean that others' attention as well as their respect will be hers.

Next, we have the 'destructive drunken lesbian'. She is a white woman who has been divorced for five years. She is 30 years old and employed in a high-status job in a legal firm. She used to drink very moderately. In fact, up until six months ago, she had not been drinking any alcohol at all for almost two years. However, for the past three months she has been drinking quite heavily — at least a half bottle of Scotch at home alone or out with friends in the evening. She has managed to hide her drinking from her workmates. She has her own office and is therefore able to keep it a secret that she suffers from daily hangovers at her workplace. She is becoming quite dependent upon alcohol and has started to admit it, but only to herself. When she gets drunk in the evening, she is quite depressed and grieving because she has just broken off a relationship with a woman she still loves deeply.

At work where she has come out as a lesbian, she acts very destructively and taunts her workmates, including her boss. She may lose her job if she continues. Her conduct has brought out destructiveness in her colleagues. Recently she has been the target of gay jokes. But she actually feels guilty about being a lesbian and frustrated that her colleagues would never understand her or her recently self-inflicted pain. She lives the life of a woman on the road to self-destruction. Her life is full of guilt, pain and self-hate.

For her, a less damaging image of herself could be a 'dignified woman'. Although this woman may go through difficult and even painful times in her life, she is able to carry herself with dignity. She is able to feel proud. At the very least, she knows that she can still feel, and most important that her lesbian feelings may not be understood by everyone she meets. Embracing this image of herself means that others may begin to see her dignity as a symbol of steadfastness, a basic human virtue. Rather than acting out in a destructive way, she becomes self-contained, allowing her previous unacceptable grief to be felt in her very bones. This conduct, rather than giving licence to others' destructive behaviour, allows others around her food for thought as well as space for their own feelings.

However, regardless of her dignity she may find that being an out lesbian in itself stirs all sorts of emotions in her workmates. Nevertheless, embracing dignity becomes a type of protection from further attack or verbal abuse. Most of all, a dignified person is allowed to be a feeling person, whatever these feelings may be. Overturning the image of the 'destructive lesbian' can mean that, at the very least, she begins to take control over her own life and her alcohol intake.

These examples show us how easy it may be for some women to live up to the labels that members of society slap onto them. In the above instances, these women need to work doubly hard to remove society's labels as well as their own. Overturning negative images is hard work. Simply, it is difficult psychological, emotional and social labour. This labour needs to be done by the women who have been labelled with the negative images of overdrinking women. This work is invisible; it goes on within the woman herself.

She needs to face these negative images; to see how she has been devalued by others as well as herself and to learn that for any woman to feel good enough is difficult and painful work. She needs to reach into herself to create her own standards and her own powerful images of herself. She needs to feel herself, no matter how painful the experience.

ALCOHOL AND PREGNANT WOMEN

Although I could discuss alcohol and pregnancy when we look at treatment, I made a conscious decision to discuss this issue in this chapter. On the one hand, I want to examine some of the negative images slapped on pregnant women who drink. On the other hand, I wanted to avoid falling into the usual trap of putting pregnant women into a box called 'unhealthy and in need of treatment'. When women are pregnant, their bodies become the official testing grounds of the medical profession. (For an interesting discussion of how pregnant women's bodies have been 'medicalised' and taken over by a predominantly male-led medical profession, see Ann Oakley, *The Captured Womb: A History of the Medical Care of Pregnant Women.*[9]) As this and other research shows, any pregnant woman is likely to be viewed as somehow sick, even though she may be perfectly healthy and have a healthy pregnancy. In this climate, pregnancy tends to be accepted more as a female illness than a normal life event for women. Women's bodies in a pregnant state have become increasingly 'pathologised', and medical interventions occur sometimes without good scientific evidence that they are necessary. In this way, women's reproductive powers are taken away from them as they become more and more defined by symptoms, syndromes and diagnoses made during the course of their pregnancies.

Medical ideology is often powerful and moralistic, upholding rules about women who are not 'normal' physically or psychologically. This ideology often stigmatises women for stepping out of line, particularly pregnant women. If a woman has an alcohol problem and she is pregnant, this complicates matters. Her body is seen as doubly sick – it has an infirmity (ie pregnancy) and an addiction to alcohol. Additionally, if she has a drinking problem, her mind may also be regarded as sick. It is important to separate out the scientific facts from the assumptions of the medical ideology in order to remove some of the guilt, shame and confusion women who drink may feel.

In recent years, there has been a growing concern about the effects of alcohol on the foetus. The term 'foetal alcohol syndrome' (FAS) was coined in 1973.[10] Thereafter, FAS became enshrined as an expression in the language of popular culture as well as a growth area in medical research. Doctors and researchers began to add up numbers of women giving birth to babies with FAS and by 1980 they observed 245 cases in the world.[11]

Overdrinking women became the most stigmatised group of pregnant women.[12] Nevertheless, there has been very little work which studies whether the growth of interest in FAS reflects a concern for a distinct, medical syndrome or a political matter – another way of extending the medical profession's control of women's bodies. For example, in the late 1980s, a medical syndrome called 'nutmeg intoxication'[13] was identified in pregnant women. Is avoiding nutmeg biscuits, sweets or candies while pregnant more important than generally assumed by pregnant women? What substance will be next on the list of prohibited substances for pregnant women?

But the main point here is that medical opinion on the use of alcohol by pregnant women is divided.[14] Research on FAS remains inconclusive.[15] In fact, one large study on drinking during pregnancy found that if pregnant women drank moderately, this neither presented any health problem nor caused foetal harm.[16] Conclusive research which suggests the possibility of foetal effects or harm during pregnancy tend to be studies on smoking.[17]

In order to show some of the confusion which exists in this area, let us look in detail at one woman's experience. She is a moderate drinker in her late twenties. She has recently given birth to a healthy baby boy. She spoke of her bewilderment about drinking alcohol when she was pregnant last year. While she was never told not to drink during her pregnancy, she wanted to develop a sensible attitude to drinking and most of all to 'be careful'. She says:

> I was never told not to drink while I was pregnant. But when you start to go to a pre-natal clinic they give you a little book and it gives you all sorts of information. Some of this information is about your health during pregnancy and your relationship to the foetus. It tells you what to eat. I remember it also said something like the research on the effects of alcohol on the foetus is still uncertain – but we would rather err on the side of safety and tell you 'Don't drink'. So I tried to be careful.

This woman received a different message from a doctor friend with whom she had lunch occasionally during her pregnancy. The information passed on to her from this doctor friend underlines the fact that medical opinion is divided on the matter. It challenged her expectations of drinking as a pregnant woman:

> I went out to lunch a couple of times with a doctor friend of mine. I emphasise doctor – a gynaecologist. Every time we went out to lunch he said to me, 'Have a glass of wine.' Then I would put on my act, 'I am a sensible mother to

be, I would not want to drink.' But he would say, 'Have a glass of wine – it will do you more good than harm.' So I did and that is my experience. I remembered then what I read in that little book I received at that time. It said, 'We recommend that you do not drink but if you do drink – do not drink more than one unit a week.' After I knew I was pregnant I had maybe one or two units a month and I was drinking wine.

This woman felt that she had a healthy attitude to alcohol during her pregnancy. However, before she actually knew she was pregnant, she had a drinking spree during the Christmas season. This experience caused her much anxiety once she discovered she was pregnant and learned of the possible effects of alcohol on the foetus.

Pregnant women tend to be advised to cut out alcohol altogether. If they do not, they may experience anxiety or confusion. In this context, another woman who had recently given birth recalled her experiences during pregnancy. She said that the messages she received about FAS were mainly from the media. The strongest message she received was that pregnant women should not drink because they were threatening the life of their future babies. She says:

The many media messages I received were to not drink during pregnancy. I tried not to drink. Even before I was pregnant I remember reading a lot in the newspapers about pregnant women and alcohol. What I read was mainly about FAS and the problems a woman will have if she drinks while she is pregnant. Basically, these articles said a pregnant woman was threatening the life of her baby if she drank. So I had heard a lot about FAS even before I got pregnant.

From the above comments, we see that women receive

powerful messages about alcohol and pregnancy. These messages, deeply embedded in our culture, attempt to control pregnant women's relationship to alcohol. As a result, if these women choose to drink, they will be the recipients of negative moral judgements. Simply, they will be made to feel guilty, ashamed and, in the end, the image of 'baby destroyers' emerges. Cavalier statements are made blaming these women for being a main cause of mental retardation in the western world.[18] The main point here is that the message 'Do not drink during pregnancy' appears to be based on unequivocal, scientific fact – which in fact it isn't.

In this moral crusade, any pregnant woman who drinks is stigmatised, while a whole body of medical literature attempts to safeguard this stigma. In addition, women are often pressurised by medical slogans: 'Don't drink during pregnancy'; 'Think of your baby before you drink'; 'Do you want a retarded child?'; 'Stop taking alcohol', and so on. Pregnant women hear these constant refrains. But what they do not hear is that FAS is linked more to the actual amount of alcohol a woman drinks than to alcohol itself. Simply, if a pregnant woman drinks heavily over long periods of time, the foetus is more at risk than if a pregnant woman drinks slightly or moderately.

In this context, it is interesting that few doctors or scientists make it known that testicle shrinkage or atrophy occurs in men who are heavy drinkers[19] and that this affects the potency of their sperm. On the whole, men drink more alcohol and more heavily than women. What doctor would dare to tell a drinking man wanting to father a child to cut out drinking altogether? This suggests that women's bodies, sexuality and drinking behaviour are in need of more control than men's. It also suggests further that FAS may be as much about increasing medical control over women's bodies during pregnancy as the prevention of foetal harm.

Clearly, the double standard raises its ugly head. The FAS is used to target pregnant women who bear children – not men who father them. The hidden message is not only that women are less responsible in their drinking than men but also that women's bodies need more control and surveillance than men's bodies. In turn, the doctor appears as the protector of the foetus and, of course, women are told that they cannot manage without the doctor. Pregnant women therefore appear as being incapable of protecting their own bodies during pregnancy.

If women were informed of the risks of *heavy* drinking during pregnancy rather than told to stop drinking altogether (and given heavy moral judgements if they don't), most women would probably take the necessary precautions and not drink heavily. This is not meant to imply that all women will stop drinking heavily, whether informed of the risks or not. Of course, some women do drink heavily, for whatever reason, and continue to do so during pregnancy. The implication here is that women need to be given a choice in this matter as well as correct information about alcohol and pregnancy, based on clear scientific evidence – not moral judgements. For example, there is a big difference between telling a pregnant woman to stop drinking totally because one sees it as morally reprehensible and telling a woman to stop drinking heavily because it is a proven medical fact that heavy drinking during pregnancy may be physically harmful to her and the foetus. Women must not be kept in a state of ignorance.

The above discussion is not meant to advocate that women drink more than moderately during pregnancy. If women drink during pregnancy, as some choose to do, they should know the risks involved. But these risks have existed for as long as alcohol has been around. On the other hand, there is a need to expose some of the hidden issues that are involved in discussions of FAS. In exposing these issues, FAS appears as a political issue, having a profound influence on many pregnant women's experiences in both the public and private spheres of their lives.

The confusing mixture of information on FAS can be a 'dangerous social cocktail' because it acts as a poison which kills a woman's right to take responsibility for her body and drinking during pregnancy. Women need to know that their well-being and that of their future children is in their own hands. One woman therapist put an interesting twist on these ideas when she said:

> Think of how often pregnant women are told not to drink during pregnancy. Many experts believe that pregnant women's drinking will destroy future children. But I have seen women who are never told or warned by their doctors to avoid physically violent husbands during pregnancy. It is men more than women's drinking alcohol that is the cause of these women's miscarriages. No one ever talks about this issue. No, they'd rather blame women.

Notes

1. Jean Kirkpatrick, 'Preface to the 1986 Edition', *Turnabout: New Help for the Woman Alcoholic* (Seattle: Madrona Publishers, 1986).
2. Dimitra Gefou-Madianou's excellent discussion of the need for an anti-domestic discourse on alcohol emphasises quite strongly this way of thinking. See Dimitra Gefou-Madianou, 'Alcohol Commensality, Identity Transformations and Transcendence' in Dimitra Gefou-Madianou, ed, *Alcohol, Gender and Culture* (New York and London: Routledge, 1992).

3. Here, Max Glatt is referring to common personality types of wives of alcoholics as proposed by an American researcher, Thelma Whalen, in 1953. See Max Glatt, *Alcoholism* (Sevenoaks, UK: Hodder and Stoughton, 1982).

4. See the classic example, M Sandmair, *The Invisible Alcoholics: Women and Alcohol Abuse in America* (New York: McGraw Hill, 1980).

5. In everyday usage, 'stereotypes' refer to the mental pictures that people can have about others in society. Often, these mental pictures are seen to be held by members of a particular social group against another group (eg Irish men like to drink, black men are lazy, and so on). In reality, stereotypes represent oversimplified beliefs, feelings or judgements of a type of person, an ethnic group, a social event, a social issue, and so on. Stereotypes can hurt. I prefer to use the word 'images' rather than 'stereotypes' throughout this chapter. This is because I want to emphasise the idea, along with Dorothy Smith, that there is often a process of the 'standardisation of images' that goes beyond mere mental pictures or moral judgements, feelings or beliefs. For example, when images of women become standardised, these images become the currency of most if not all social interpretations and become deeply rooted in the minds of those who create the images. Images are more powerful weapons against women than stereotypes. Examining these can help us to see more clearly the process behind how women are judged in everyday life. See Dorothy Smith, *Texts, Facts and Femininity: Exploring the Relations of Ruling* (London: Routledge, 1990), especially Chapter 6, 'Femininity as discourse', pp 159–208.

6. See another classic, K M Fillmore, 'When Angels Fall: Women's Drinking as Cultural Preoccupation and as Reality', in SC Wilsnack and L Beckman, eds, *Alcohol Problems in Women: Antecedents and Consequences* (New York: Guilford Press, 1984).

7. One of the earliest classics in this area is J Harwin and S Otto, 'Women, Alcohol and the Screen', in J Cook and M Lewington, eds, *Images of Alcoholism* (London: British Film Institute and Alcohol Education Centre, 1979). It is an excellent account of the images of women drinkers on screen.

8. As in earlier discussions in this book, the stories that follow are based on true stories of women who experienced negative drinking. Here, I give as much detail as I can about their personal lives while still protecting their anonymity.

9. Ann Oakley, *The Captured Womb: A History of the Medical Care of*

Pregnant Women (Oxford: Basil Blackwell, 1984).

10. See KL Jones and DW Smith, 'Recognition of the Foetal Alcohol Syndrome in Early Infancy', *Lancet* 2 (1973): 999–1001.

11. See HL Rosett, 'The Effects of Alcohol on the Fetus and Offspring' in OJ Kalant, ed, *Alcohol and Drug Problems in Women* (New York and London: Plenum Press, 1980).

12. Also, cocaine-using women giving birth to 'crack babies' could be considered a related stigmatised group. See, for example, G Walker, Kathleen Eric, A Pivnick and E Drucker, 'A Descriptive Outline of a Program for Cocaine-using Mothers and their Babies' in Claudio Bepko, ed, *Feminism and Addiction* (New York, London and Sydney: Haworth Press, 1991).

13. See G Lauy, 'Nutmeg Intoxication in Pregnancy: A Case Report', *Journal of Reproductive Medicine* 32, 1 (1987): 63–64.

14. Alcohol Concern, *Women and Drinking* (London: Alcohol Concern, 1988).

15. While Nancy Day notes that the relationship between exposure to alcohol and the degree of foetal effect is not clear, she nevertheless is a firm believer in FAS. See Nancy L Day, 'The Effects of Prenatal Exposure to Alcohol' in *Alcohol World and Health Research* 10 (1992): 3.

16. See Moira Plant, *Women, Drinking and Pregnancy* (London: Tavistock, 1985), in which she reports that 'moderate' levels of drinking during pregnancy means fewer than 10 units of alcohol per week (1 unit is the equivalent of a 4 oz. or 120ml glass of wine).

17. The earliest evidence of the effects of smoking on women's reproductive processes appeared in 1935. See LN Sontage and RF Wallace, 'The Effect of Smoking During Pregnancy on the Fetal Heart Rate', *American Journal of Obstetrics and Gynecology* 29 (1935): 77–83.

18. Nancy Day, in 'The Effects of Prenatal Exposure to Alcohol', notes that 'FAS is one of the commonest causes of mental retardation', and this sentence is repeated almost verbatim by Katherine van Wormer, *Alcoholism Treatment: A Social Work Perspective* (Chicago: Nelson Hall Publishers, 1995), p 99, demonstrating that even gender-sensitive researchers or feminists can take the 'FAS hook'.

19. This is an issue that is discussed in I Robertson and N Heather, *Let's Drink to Your Health* (Leicester: British Psychological Society, 1986).

CHAPTER 4

Female 'treatment' or women-healing?

INTRODUCTION

It is hard to count how many years I have worked in this
field because it's been such a long time. My first job was
in an alcohol agency and I worked with both men and
women. It was hard at first . . . especially to work with
women . . . but it was very interesting . . . I found there
wasn't any history or any knowledge about women to lean
on. It was such a hidden area.

This woman summed up her experiences working as a
professional counsellor in an alcohol treatment agency. Over
the years, she has run women-only groups and has gained
much experience in this area. She enjoys working with
women because this work has provided her with insights
into how women deal with their problems of living and,
specifically, helped her to understand some of the reasons
why women overdrink. For her, helping women was 'a
hidden area' and this hiddenness made it more difficult to
work with women than she had thought initially.

With these ideas in mind, let us focus more closely on the
alcohol treatment industry, which has become a lucrative
business in the field of addiction treatment.[1] This is mainly

because in richer countries the alcohol industry is highly profitable. In many alcohol agencies throughout Europe and the United States, the emphasis is on producing a cure. The end product is the 'cured alcoholic', who may pay vast amounts of money to those willing to sell him/her this cure.

In this context, I want to re-emphasise a key problem which I noted earlier in the Introduction: women already in the treatment system or those seeking 'official' help tend to be looked upon as representative of all women overdrinkers. In this chapter, I want to explore the complexities of this problem because, when we look beyond the field of alcohol treatment, we find that the psychology of women's overdrinking is different from the male variety;[2] and recovering from overdrinking for many women is really about recovering from female socialisation – and requires that a woman learn to care about her relationship to herself as she cares about her relationships with others.[3] This type of recovery process does not necessarily demand entry into an official treatment system.

Thus, that women in treatment or seeking treatment have been viewed by alcohol experts as representative of most, if not all, women with drinking problems has put undue emphasis upon the lives, experiences and problems of these women. In fact, the experiences of women overdrinkers who *don't* seek official treatment might be very different. Additionally, there is a hidden assumption operating behind the expert's view: if women overdrink, they should be in official treatment. There is a need to look beyond treatment settings to gain a richer view of women who neither fit into this traditional picture nor warrant this type of treatment. Some women do not seek nor want such treatment.

One woman who experienced negative drinking (ie overdrinking) but not alcohol treatment, is concerned that men and women are judged differently in relation to drinking. She believes that a moralistic double standard governing men's and women's drinking behaviour exists in society and is mirrored in official treatment settings, where it is used to evaluate men and women coming forward for help. Her implication is that treaters provide the 'treatment' rules that are based on stereotypes of how men and women should and should not drink. But these treaters believe that men and women drink for the same reasons; they fail to see the differences in why men and women drink:

> Women are not free to choose the ways in which they drink. Women don't start drinking from the same position as men [in wider society].

Now, I would like to begin building a new vision of how women experience a need for alcohol 'treatment'. In my experience of working with women who have problems with all sorts of substances, including alcohol,[4] I have found that, regardless of whether or not they seek treatment, they urgently need to experience compassion from others as well as humane help. I emphasise that women are usually seeking 'help' rather than 'treatment'. 'Help' is also a more familiar and 'user friendly' word than 'treatment'. Help, received and given, is an everyday fact of life. Often, we need help and we seek help because we hurt. Help implies human agency: we help ourselves and others, and others help us. In this context, we may perhaps experience physical, personal and social damage, or deep wounding, due to our overdrinking. The fact that we are women compounds matters. Being less than 'real' women (ie morally sub-standard or 'fallen women'[5]) makes it even more difficult for us to seek help, to repair our damage and to heal our wounds.

This type of viewpoint differs in many ways from traditions existing in the alcohol field. This is because the majority of alcohol treatment professionals focus on what they call the 'treatment of female alcoholics'.[6] The alternative view, which is put forward here, highlights the need to speak about women-helping and women-healing more than the 'treatment of female alcoholics'. This alternative way of speaking is miles, perhaps light years, away from the traditional way of speaking about women in the alcohol field. While this women-healing or helping view began to gain visibility in the early 1980s,[7] it remains a minority view and offers a non-traditional as well as an 'unofficial' way of seeing women who experience alcohol problems.

This women-healing view may appear as a secondary one because, at heart, it offers a view from 'below' – from the hidden vista of women who more often than not appear as secondary to men. When women's overdrinking becomes visible in treatment settings, the needs of women appear minor compared to men's. As we have seen, overdrinking women are seen as inferior, as 'damaged goods', in contrast to their male counterparts and often in comparison to other 'normal' women (ie those who do not overdrink), and stereotypes which abound in the wider world often also apply in official treatment settings.

A sense of urgency comes with the need to build a view of healing and helping based on women's needs and experiences. No woman with a drinking problem needs more damage. She has already experienced enough physical, psychological and social damage due to overdrinking. But a basic fact of life is that for some women treatment causes further damage. This is why we need to be aware of the official view of the 'treatment of female alcoholics'[8] based on the needs and experiences of experts, treaters, researchers or those apparently 'in the know', while, at the same time, speak loudly and clearly about the need for women-healing. For example, women aproaching treatment need to take precautions to protect themselves from further harm in treatment. It is good practice to get a clear look at treatment programmes before committing to one. People, particularly women, entering a treatment programme can be very vulnerable. They need to enter treatment with their eyes wide open. This is an issue which will be discussed further in the following chapter.

To construct an alternative, women-healing view is to actively create a gender-sensitive viewpoint, challenging the idea of 'female treatment', based on the whims, gendered ideologies and powerful discourses of those 'in the know'. A gender-sensitive viewpoint is shaped by the artistry of healing – a craft developed out of the real, human experiences and needs of damaged, wounded and discarded women. Within this viewpoint, healing is an empowering process as well as an experience that generates strength and self-worth rather than fear, guilt, shame and further wounding.

Before we disengage ourselves from the idea of treatment and embrace the concept of healing, let us ask ourselves two key questions: What is meant by treatment? and How are women 'treated' by treatment?

WHAT IS MEANT BY TREATMENT?

In general parlance, the word 'treatment' refers to the method of dealing with or behaving towards a person or a thing. For example, one says, 'She was given rough treatment by her boyfriend/girlfriend', 'The doctor said she must follow the prescribed treatment' or 'The wooden table is now ready for treatment with varnish'. Here, 'treatment' refers to a way of handling or dealing with someone or something – in the above cases – a young woman, a female patient and a wooden table.

In the alcohol field, 'treatment' refers to the way of treating, dealing with, managing and handling the alcoholic, this 'someone' who has a problem with drinking. My main point, here, is that regardless of who receives or provides treatment or how it is received or given, treatment is all about *doing something to change someone*. The agent of change (ie the treater) is not the same person who actually needs the experience of change (ie the treated). In this view, treatment is about managing and handling someone needing correction and change because this someone cannot 'handle' their alcohol.[9] But, in this 'doing something to change someone', too much emphasis can be placed upon external factors such as the methods of treatment or treatment regimes, devised by the treater, rather than on the internal factor of healing needed by the one being treated.

For example, treaters develop methods of getting the alcoholic to change her/his behaviour in a variety of treatment regimes. But implicit in these treatment methods is the idea that the treated cannot be her/his own agent of change without the help of the treater. In the end, the needs of the treater to provide good treatment may take priority over the needs of the treated – the actual person in need of help. In this way, the treated, experiencing traditional forms of treatment, may appear as somewhat passive or at least as less active than the treater.

Of course, whoever does the 'doing' – the alcohol treating – is more often than not the person with the most power, influence and control in the treatment situation. Thus a picture emerges: the treater, offering the 'cure', rather than the treated receiving the 'cure', knows best. There is a deep and hidden moral claim being made here: 'The one who knows best gives best', and this type of claim sets up an unnecessary hierarchy in treatment establishments.

While most, if not all, treatment establishments operate on this basis, this system of ranking the treater on a higher moral level than the treated tends to remain invisible and can be damaging to the treatment process. This invisible hierarchy is not only about who has the most power in treatment situations but also about who holds knowledge of the 'cure'. Unfortunately, when mixed with gender inequalities, this hierarchy can make treatment uncomfortable for women.

HOW ARE WOMEN 'TREATED' BY TREATMENT?[10]

Regardless of whether or not women seek treatment, they often receive powerful messages from their treaters such as: 'You should stop drinking', 'You are hurting yourself', 'You are a pathological liar', 'You must learn self-control', 'You need to count your alcohol units', 'You need to do a drinking diary', 'You need to fill in the alcohol dependence questionnaire', 'You need electric shock treatment', 'You need an employee assistance programme', 'You need intensive psychotherapy', 'You need detoxification', 'You need group work', 'You need psychoanalysis', 'You need relaxation training', 'You need an in-patient programme', 'You need day-patient treatment'; 'You need these pills',[11] 'You need a recovery regime' and so on. For any woman seeking treatment, these messages may appear endless.

Often, the hidden messages are even more powerful: 'You are a disgrace', 'You're a hopeless case', 'You are contemptible', 'You are a bad mother', 'You are worthless', 'You should be ashamed of yourself', 'You're neglecting your family', 'You should feel guilty', 'You are unfeminine', 'You are a drunk', etc. All of these messages, whether spoken or unspoken, can be heard by women who seek treatment. These messages tend to be created by treaters who believe, 'I know what's best for her and she needs treatment'.

WOMEN-HEALING

We rarely hear treaters ask an overdrinking woman: 'Would

you like to learn about giving up overdrinking and strengthen your female self?' 'Would you like to learn how to transform your shame into self-love?' 'Would you like to have another friend besides alcohol?' 'Would you like understanding?' and 'Would you like to feel less lost in your life?'

These sorts of questions encourage a humane, compassionate and benevolent response. They allow any woman to give mercy to herself. They convey clear, strong messages which a wounded woman needs to hear: 'You have worth', 'You can learn the art of self-healing', 'You can learn to empower yourself as a woman', 'You can face your difficult and painful feelings' and 'You can accept yourself even though you experience negative drinking – in contrast to the destructive messages of many treaters. As non-invading, respectful and sincere, these questions uphold the integrity of the person who is asking the question as well as the woman to whom the question is being asked.

To begin to answer these empowering questions in this study of treatment is to begin to move onto a different plane and to create a new quality of response. This new quality of response can be found in the area of healing – women-healing. As we now disengage ourselves from the traditional views of treating women, we will look at the importance of each of the above-mentioned questions. In our attempt to build an alternative picture of 'treatment' for women, our canvas is shaped by an understanding of healing, as we hear the voices of women's experiences.

Would you like to learn about giving up overdrinking and strengthen your female self?

One woman who called herself an 'ex-alcoholic' spoke about her own process of self-healing. She told about how she had to remember and to regain lost parts of her self, as she went through this process. With her own eyes, she saw how she had 'given up' herself through drinking:

> Your self, in a way, is taken from you when you drink and you find that you give yourself up in the face of alcohol. So for me, I had to actually remember and take those parts of myself back – whatever it was that I gave up through drink. Somehow, I had to learn to turn that whole thing around.

In describing this very intimate and painful process, she spoke about her ideas on how women can experience their own 'recoveries' in very positive and powerful ways. In her opinion, it was easier for women to recover than men:

> Women do not have the severe problem with humility that men do. To recover you need to surrender – somehow to give up. You need to accept the way that you are and what you have done and who you are. Of course, this hurts. But we women have not been taught to think that much of ourselves. In a way, that is our salvation because it means that in some ways we are allowed to be humble with ourselves.

For this woman, to be humble is a key with which to awaken the beginnings of a sense of oneself. Humility allowed her to accept herself and her drinking. In the end, being humble allowed her to identify with overdrinking and, in turn, to give it up. In her view, women are able to bear the depth of this humility: they make 'tremendous growth' on a 'qualitative level'. However, this process is not easy:

> It is terrible and very painful to actually say, 'I identify with alcohol. This is what I am addicted to.' You need to be very humble. I – myself – me – I am willing to give it up. I am willing to transcend those depths.

On the other hand, she believed that for a man to 'transcend those depths' was a different story. While women could be enriched by the spirit of humility, men appear to fight it. Here, she had an interesting insight:

A man fights with this spirit of humility. It is anathema to him. He hates it. 'How can I surrender to that image of myself?' he asks. It is totally alien to men – totally emasculating. A man asks, 'How am I going to view myself?' . . . That there is an area in life where he does not have it all set up and done for him somehow shakes him up . . .

Obviously, this woman sees differences in the ways women and men go through the process of healing. While masculinity could interfere with a man's healing process, femininity, which carries less social value, could actually work to a woman's advantage. The reason she gave was that women have less trouble than men in experiencing humility.

The point is that humility makes it easier to sense that one needs to change one's life and face oneself. Humility is an asset rather than a liability. So for this woman, it was possible with humility to make tremendous growth in facing an alcohol problem as well as to strengthen her female self. This implies that women need 'to turn around' what has been traditionally seen as female weakness and make it one's strength. She continues:

You see what actually devalues women in society may actually save them in addiction. They do not have this great inflated idea of themselves – this great big ego. So women can give up alcohol more easily than men. They can heal themselves.

Would you like to learn how to transform your shame into self-love?

Most if not all of the overdrinking women with whom I have spoken pinpoint a deep feeling of shame. This sense of shame is all about bearing overdrinking as a heavy social burden – as a very real way of going against society's and others' ideas of what it means to be an acceptable woman. A woman feels guilt and shame, and at times these feelings are unbearable. They generate further a deep self-loathing and can block a sense of self-love.

One woman counsellor described how a woman's experience of shame helps to fuel denial. Simply, a woman full of shame denies that she is overdrinking. Shame is able to block a sense of reality and oneself. She said:

> If a woman's drinking has been a problem, she may not recognise it as her problem. There is always this denial. Women refuse they have a problem. This is how I see it. I see it from a woman, when I ask her about alcohol. Then there is denial. I always sense it from the first question. If I ask, 'Do you drink alcohol?', I get interesting answers such as 'Yeah, but I have always done my work' or 'Yes, everybody drinks'. When a woman answers in this way, I say to myself, 'Why doesn't she just say that I drink two glasses of wine a day?' But I know she can't. She's in denial. You hear the denial from the answer.

Besides seeing 'denial', this woman counsellor also talked about the ways she sensed women's shame. She believes that women are unable to really heal themselves and stop overdrinking without 'overcoming their shame'. In her work she tries to sense whether or not a woman carries, what she calls, the 'smell' of alcohol. This 'smell' is not the actual alcohol fumes coming from one's mouth but a 'kind of emotional smell'. Usually she 'smells alcohol' when she encounters a woman's silence. This happens when she asks about alcohol and receives a 'silent answer'. In her view, much is spoken in women's silence:

> With women there can be this deep, dreadful silence. For me, it almost smells like death. It is like a big, big shame. Then, I sense that a woman does not want to talk about it or rather can't even talk about it. It is so forbidden to her. If a woman can't talk about alcohol like a natural thing, then I see in my mind a yellow light blinking. 'Ah ha!'; 'I think she has some problem with alcohol'; or 'She has a problem', I say to myself. Then, there is this silence. I just hear the silence. It means to me a silence which is almost too deep. It is either this silent shame or a type of denial that includes a lot of explanations, like everybody is doing it [drinking a lot], it's not just me.

For any overdrinking woman, dipping into oneself can be a painful process. Nevertheless, to overcome the 'smell like death' or the 'big, big shame' in one's life is to learn to accept oneself. But healing and self-love can only take place in the alcoholic wound itself: if the woman is prepared to travel into the wound; to examine why she is drinking, what she is like when she is drinking, and what part of herself she is losing. In this context, I recall the penetrating words of one woman. We were sitting in her home. She was telling me about her experience of recovering from alcohol after a six-year 'destructive bout with alcohol'. Over our cups of tea, she said:

> You can only heal yourself and truly recover if you face yourself – take a good look at yourself. And that means finding some – any piece of self-love, anything you can find to get over the contempt – the hate – the denial of the good you have in yourself.

For this woman, I 'smelled' her self-love, but a love, I thought at that moment, gained by entering her self-inflicted wound of overdrinking.

Would you like to have another friend besides alcohol?

Very often women refer to alcohol as 'my best friend'. I asked one woman who has been a member of AA for 21 years what was the most frequent symbol that women use with alcohol. In response, she said what came immediately into her mind, 'Alcohol is my friend.' She then described her own personal experience concerning the idea that 'alcohol is my friend'. First, she talked about her own 'friendship' relationship with alcohol. She said:

> I grew up being very self-sufficient, self-contained, and very frightened. Initially, I encountered alcohol in social situations around the age of 16. That is really where I met alcohol. I said to myself; 'This is my friend' and 'This is terrific'. Alcohol was my friend. I did not mean it in any special context, only that alcohol makes me feel OK. It relaxes me. I can be amusing and funny and I do not need to be afraid. You see alcohol takes away all of my inhibitions and I have a good time. I could be the life of the party. I was probably disappearing halfway through the party in order to go outside and get sick in the bushes. But at the time, I was building up a tolerance for alcohol. So that is how I came to describe alcohol as my friend.

In her view, the idea that 'alcohol is my friend' was really a false idea by which she had deluded herself. At first, she thought this friend was worthy of her trust, but in the end alcohol did not merit her trust.

> I drank from the age of 16 until I was 33. But alcohol was definitely a friend I could trust. Of course, I thought this,

but this is always the illusion with alcohol. If I wanted company or to be with someone, I only had to have my bottle. Even if I was in a social situation, alcohol could put the needed distance between me and others. And I thought I had control over my friend.

She stressed that alcohol had been her friend in helping her cope with loneliness and hurt. But this friendship gradually backfired. Alcohol became her worst enemy, causing much trouble and hardship:

If I had been offended or upset in any way, I could go and have a drink and that would make it all right. So a man or a woman could offend me, but not alcohol – it was my friend. Of course, when alcohol stopped being my friend and made trouble, I still did not realise it was hurting me. I could not see the reason why I was getting into trouble and ending up in strange beds. It is amazing. I never got raped; I never got pregnant; I never got robbed; I never got mugged. I was very lucky because I had been in situations which when I think back on them today, I absolutely shudder. I never made the connection between my troubles and alcohol. I never said to myself, 'I am getting into trouble because alcohol is my friend.'

She then focused her attention on her experiences with other women in AA meetings and how these women's experiences matched hers. She has participated in many AA women's meetings:

If you go to these meetings and listen to what these women are saying, you always hear 'alcohol is my friend.' It took time for me to realise, 'Hey, these women's lives are like mine!'

She continues:

I heard 'alcohol is my friend' said many times. Women say they are loners. I think when you say you are a loner it creates a circle of isolation. If you are isolated to begin with, then you can become a drunk. It is like two walls of defence. So when I came into AA, I heard many women talking about being loners and self-sufficient: 'I don't need any help', or 'Never mind, I can do this myself.' I heard that kind of attitude and arrogance. Then I thought, 'Yes, I can identify with this.' I was hearing a lot of the same things I was feeling from other women.

For this woman, the 'alcohol is my friend' idea creates a circle of isolation. Women must face up to experiences of themselves as lonely, while at the same time accepting that they have a destructive relationship with alcohol. As was the case with this woman, facing up to herself became easier the more she heard other women with similar experiences. However, these experiences were, at times, devastating and unforgivable:

There are a lot of women who cannot forgive themselves for having put themselves into unthinkable situations. It is very hard for them. I think that if a woman has been raped and has an alcohol problem on top of that, it must be devastating. You really are [devastated]. You hear a lot of this from women who are raped. Then the tears start and 'I was raped as a child' or 'I was abused by my father' and on and on. Having to live with that devastation, women medicate with alcohol to remove the pain.

This woman understood why, in particular, women who were victims of abuse from others would see alcohol as their friend. She believed this was a meaningful metaphor, matching their experiences. In the midst of abuse, they needed a friend to rely on, and alcohol was the only friend there for them. She says:

If abused women medicate with alcohol, it numbs them so that they can cope. 'Alcohol is my friend' becomes a very meaningful metaphor in that kind of context.

The idea of alcohol as a friend provides valuable insights. It demonstrates that while most if not all of us have the need for companionship and friendship, those who overdrink fulfil this need through alcohol. Understanding the metaphor 'alcohol is my friend' enables us to see that women need to forgive themselves for their destructive friendship with alcohol; women need to move beyond finding their need for friendship 'in a bottle'; and women need a symbol that actually matches their experiences (ie an abused woman needs a real friend).

Surprisingly, this metaphor may help abused and self-abusing women to put their feelings into a worthwhile context. For example, using this metaphor may provide an overdrinking woman with a challenging insight: 'I need a real, human friend.' When this 'friend' can be found in herself or others, she may discover that she no longer needs to medicate her loneliness, pain, anguish, hurt or despair through her 'bottled, non-human friend', alcohol.

As we see, the metaphor 'alcohol is my friend' has the potential to be a positive symbol in restoring physical and emotional well-being, if women are able to break from the destructive power of alcohol. This is because the notion of friendship is transformative and healing for women,[12] allowing them to recognise and begin to mend wounds. Every woman needs a friend; but at times we feel the need to reject a friend for our own good because this friend doesn't stop hurting us. Healing our negative drinking is all about 'saying no' to this kind of hurt.

Would you like understanding?

This next question relates to an important conversation I had with an alcohol therapist. She believes strongly that women who overdrink need understanding. For her, understanding is a key for both a woman and her helper, viewed as someone 'who gains knowledge of a woman's overdrinking'. On the one hand, a woman begins healing by knowing that her life lacks understanding. On the other hand, a helper finds out the reasons why it is 'understandable' that women drink too much.

If a woman is constantly drinking for emotional or psychological reasons, then it can be that she cannot cope with her feelings. She finds that she is always lacking something – understanding. When the helper as the other person sees this, she needs to explore what she sees and to think 'Yes, it is very understandable that "so and so" drinks'.

Let us focus for a moment on this other person, the helper, rather than the woman drinker. The mere fact that this 'other' finds within herself/himself the reasons why it is understandable that a woman overdrinks can generate a powerful healing process. Simply, it can be a way of bestowing the precious gift of understanding upon the woman who overdrinks. It is saying in a very strong way, 'I accept you and your pain, regardless of how you have coped with your pain.'

In this way, the healing process can begin because the need for understanding is recognised and the seed of self-love can start to grow within the overdrinker. As stated earlier, the concept of healing tends to remain outside of the traditional alcohol treatment picture. Additionally, the conception of learning the craft of self-love and self-worth is also missing.

When treatment is about doing something to the treated, the person who is trying to help (ie the treater) has a tendency to be unable to understand why women are overdrinking. As a result, she/he cannot really give appropriate help. 'Doing something' to the treated is very different from giving the gift of understanding to those women in need of self-healing.

Would you like to feel less lost in your life?

In my experience within alcohol treatment establishments, I have heard many women speak about their deep sense of feeling lost. For example, I have heard: 'I have no aim in my life'; 'I am lost within myself'; 'I am a lost soul'; 'I have not found hope in my life'; 'I am losing the grip I once had on my life'; 'I wish I did not feel so hopeless and lost – I do not know what to do'; and so on.

Perhaps the above comments seem a bit exaggerated. You may ask, 'What does alcohol have to do with these feelings?' But this is the reality of some women's lives. The expression 'to lose yourself in a bottle' is actually quite appropriate, especially for women. It is, in my view, very understandable that apparently damaged, second-rate or devalued individuals lacking self-esteem would lose themselves or even want to lose themselves in a bottle. While a woman may not drink all of the time, she may find that as an overdrinker she is plagued either by feeling lost or by actually experiencing being lost in her social world.

Feelings of being lost have a direct impact on a woman overdrinker's day-to-day life. Not only is she lost from herself and feels this at a very deep level but also she may experience being lost from her sense of time and place. But, before we study how one loses a sense of time and place, we should look briefly at how alcohol actually causes memory loss and 'blackouts'. I describe this process through the words of one older woman and I see this story as quite instructive – particularly for younger women, who should be aware that alcohol does not discriminate by age.

This older woman is around 65 years old. She had been a very heavy spirits drinker when she was younger. About 10 years ago, she stopped drinking spirits altogether but still drank wine. She came from an upper-class family and socialised in a similar group of friends before she went to university. She recalled an alarming occurrence from her youth. After many years, the experience was still an important one:

> I was about 18 years old and I remember it was the summer time. I was with friends and we wanted to have a picnic. We spent a long day together eating and drinking. Some friends were playing tennis. Somebody gave me a bottle of alcohol to drink; I just washed it down. But, bang, it was strong stuff. I found out later it was pure alcohol. I do not know where my friend got it and the strange thing is that I do not know what happened after that. All I remember is that we all went somewhere that evening, then my mind goes blank. I was told by one friend that I actually drove all of us home later on in the evening. But, you know, to this day I do not remember how I did it. I have a total memory loss. It was kind of scary but it must have been the alcohol. I was young then and did not know about any of these things – it was just a joke. But I lost a whole day of my life.

This is an extreme case because pure alcohol was involved, but this woman's experience does emphasise that alcohol can cause severe memory losses or blackouts which are usually good indications of a severe alcohol problem.[13]

Regardless of whether or not those who overdrink experience such severe memory losses, they will inevitably find that alcohol makes them feel lost in their lives or that it is hard to 'keep promises' around time. For instance, many overdrinkers find it difficult to be on time for an appointment or a meeting – with a friend, a doctor, a mother, a relative, etc. One lesbian spoke about how her friend, another lesbian, had an alcohol problem. She started to see this as a problem because her friend was 'chronically late' for everything that they had planned together:

> I found out that she was an alcoholic at the time. Once she invited me to her home. We were going to do some redecorating together. We planned to meet at a certain time on the weekend. After she invited me there, she was not home. It was awful. I could not believe it, but this was always happening.

Another woman, a therapist, spoke about her experience with some of her women clients. It was difficult for them to be on time for appointments; they would make an arrangement to meet and then not show up:

> You find out with women who have an alcohol problem that it is very hard for them to be on time. If a woman cannot remember what she has to do and when, she has a problem. The first thing I think is that she is using alcohol and is acting out. Being late means that she is using alcohol and needs to act out in her life. Alcohol is a good way to act out. It is a good excuse. You can behave badly and blame alcohol – even though you may not even be drinking alcohol at that moment. Usually, this is because as a drinker you are not so aware of time or of your emotions and behaviour.

The above therapist also gave an example of how losing a sense of time and space was linked to expressing shame and guilt for overdrinking women. She spoke about one such woman she had seen recently:

> [Name of woman] could never come to my session on time. I do not mean to say that she didn't come because she was drinking or even drunk. But I would say that her not coming on time was all about her guilt and shame about drinking. This was why she could not come to meet me . . . She was guilty and ashamed. And I found this out from her. She told me that she was feeling more and more ashamed of her drinking.

Later on in our discussion, this therapist spoke about how losing a sense of time reflected deep lost feelings – a key to understanding a woman's problems. She believes that a woman creates a type of 'feeling lost' attitude and that this attitude influences her entire life.

> The idea of time is very important. These women lose time. They have lost time – the sense of time. They are lost in every way. They are lost from time and place and from themselves . . . This becomes a type of attitude.

These words may create an image of a lost or forlorn woman or a woman with nowhere to go in life. Alcohol may have shown the way to go, but after a while it doesn't and it can't. It causes only trouble and turmoil: one loses a sense of direction. As a result, women overdrinkers experience a need for healing. However, to begin the healing process, a woman finds that she is at a loss: she is a 'double loser' because she loses her friend, alcohol, and senses at some level that she has already lost herself.

Both experiences, finding alcohol a destructive part of one's life and losing oneself through drink, cause women to feel deep shame. When the healing process gets underway, a woman finds that a sense of oneself is based simply on knowing where she is in her life. Nurturing this sense of self is about looking inwards. It is about searching for mercy and self-forgiveness, gifts which are difficult for overdrinkers to give to themselves.

Some women sense that with alcohol as a friend they looked outwards for healing, a temporary healing provided from a bottle. Perhaps they did not know how to begin the healing process – how to stop feeling lost. If women are able to develop the skill of self-healing, they find quickly that it is natural for any person to feel lost in their life. Alcohol compounds lost feelings. But the key is acceptance, not panic. Women-healing is learning how to experience lost feelings without feeling totally lost. It is all about finding that there can be a 'richness in the poverty' of lost feelings. Therefore, women do not need to try to get rid of lost feelings, they just need to learn from them.

This type of healing is most definitely a difficult process for women to go through. This is because women have not been taught how to rescue themselves. On the contrary, deeply embedded in a woman's psyche is an image of a Prince or Princess Charming rescuing her from a lost forest into which she has strayed. Rarely in the treatment process do we have images of strong women capable of or even wanting to deliver ourselves – our very own selves – from those forbidden places where we have led ourselves astray. These images have yet to be created in the world of alcohol treatment. Nevertheless, my suspicion is that a focus on the concept of women-healing should help to create new, empowering images for women.

In conclusion, this chapter has looked behind traditional ideas on female treatment and focused on women-helping and women-healing as a way of discarding damaging attitudes, images and treatment of women overdrinkers. A view of treatment based on the needs and experiences of those in the know has been discarded. We have heard the words of women speaking about healing and we have asked a series of compassionate questions. Hopefully, the profound difference between healing and treatment can be seen clearly. In the next chapter, we will continue our study of healing and look at the need for women-only services as well as women-sensitive self-help groups.

Notes

1. When I refer to 'treatment' in this chapter, I am speaking of 'official', private or state-sponsored treatment given in alcohol-treatment services, agencies, clinics, etc. I am not speaking about help received through self-help groups, such as AA. We will look at self-help in more detail in Chapter Five.

2. Katherine van Wormer, *Alcoholism Treatment: A Social Work Perspective* (Chicago: Nelson Hall Publishers, 1995), p 168.

3. J Krestan and Claudia Bepko, 'Codependency: The Social Reconstruction of Female Experience', in Claudia Bepko, ed, *Feminism and Addiction* (New York, London and Sydney: The Haworth Press, 1991).

4. For insights into women's use of substances besides alcohol, see Elizabeth Ettorre, *Women and Substance Use* (London: Macmillan and New Brunswick, NJ: Rutgers University Press, 1992).

5. Lesley Doyal, *What Makes Women Sick* (London: Macmillan, 1995), p 180.

6. Margaret Sargent refers to traditional treatment as 'conventional intervention' and argues that 'conventional forms of intervention perpetuate the inequality of women'. See Margaret Sargent, *Women, Drugs and Policy in Sydney, London and Amsterdam* (Aldershot, UK: Avebury Press, 1992), pp 202–04.

7. See, for example, Camberwell Council on Alcoholism, Women and Alcohol (London and New York: Tavistock 1980); Sheila Ernst and Lucy Goodison, *In Our Own Hands: A Book of Self-Help Therapy* (London: The Women's Press, 1981); and Bridgid McConville, *Women Under the Influence: Alcohol and its Impact* (New York: Schocken Books. 1983).

8. I would like to make it very clear here that I am not opposed to treatment. Those types of treatment which consider the needs of women who are being treated can be very helpful. For example, a woman whose body is full of alcohol to a toxic or poisonous level may not only benefit from but also urgently need detoxification in hospital. But, before she goes into hospital, she should be reassured that she will have satisfactory support as a woman during detoxification. Another woman may want to enter a group treatment programme for women with drink problems at the local alcohol clinic. She should find out what the treatment staff's views of women are.

9. Treaters tend to underemphasise the fact that this substance, alcohol, is a socially accepted and legal drug.

10. For an excellent gender-sensitive criticism of traditional treatment, see P Pasick and C White, 'Challenging General Patton: A Feminist Stance in Substance Abuse Treatment and Training' in Claudia Bepko, ed, *Feminism and Addiction*, pp 87–102.

11. Like alcohol, tranquillisers and sleeping pills can be physically addictive.

12. See Stephanie Dowrick, *The Intimacy and Solitude Self-Therapy Book* (London: The Women's Press, 1993); and Janice Raymond, *A Passion for Friends: Toward a Philosophy of Female Affection* (London: The Women's Press, 1986).

13. Katherine Van Wormer, *Alcoholism Treatment*, pp 84–85.

CHAPTER 5

Becoming strong: women-sensitivity and self-help

TREATMENT 'WORTH ITS SALT' IS WOMEN-SENSITIVE

Women alcoholics are very often put into a Catch-22 situation. If we drink, we are seen as emotional weaklings, and when we stop, many of us begin to get strong. We develop our strength as women. But a strong woman is not the norm. So often in recovery what happens is that we find ourselves back where we started – with a negative label. This label is no longer the alcoholic woman but the strong woman.

As we have seen in previous chapters, women's overdrinking can be a result of factors relating to gender. It is important therefore that any treatment or healing that takes place recognises this and has a women-sensitive treatment or healing programme.

This chapter begins by looking briefly at the need for women-sensitive services and then at women's experiences with self-help in the alcohol field. If women are going to heal themselves, they need to allow themselves to become strong. They need to develop strength, regardless of whether or not their ideas of what it means to be strong differ. A study of what makes women strong should allow women who have problems with alcohol to make more choices for themselves but, more important, to know clearly what these choices are.

In the Introduction, it was suggested that four problems need to be overcome before a women-sensitive approach is developed in the alcohol field. In discussing these problems, I noted that there is a lack of openness towards developing services catering to the needs of women and particularly towards developing women-only services, and that this lack of openness is related to a general lack of understanding about women's experiences of drinking. When we looked in detail at the official treatment world in the previous chapter, we saw how lacking official treatment is in catering to the specific needs of women. For whatever reason, however, some women may want to enter a treatment programme: they feel more secure in an organized, medical setting; they feel the need for physical care – to be actually taken care of by others; they have been drinking very heavily lately and want to be detoxified in a centre where doctors and nurses are on call to provide medical support; or they have been isolated because of drinking and do not know of any other helping agencies besides an established treatment programme.

Perhaps the official treatment programme is a local alcohol agency, which has both male and female clientele. Perhaps a woman friend found the treatment offered there helpful. Perhaps in this local agency a woman client/patient/customer can not only choose to have a woman counsellor or therapist but also select her counsellor or therapist from a group of qualified women. Perhaps, when visiting this agency and meeting staff, a woman finds that she is treated with respect and empathy. Perhaps this agency has a women-only group and this group is advertised widely in the local community. Perhaps a woman knows of someone else treated by this agency. As one woman said:

> A woman who I met in my Friday evening course at the local school attended this group and she is quite nice and is recovering. So it can't be all that bad.

Here, it is important to be aware that not all treatment programmes are run on traditional lines. While some treatments can be harmful and continue to devalue women, not all treatment is deleterious or damaging. Some treatment agencies are better for women than others; perhaps their staff tend to have more creative, women-sensitive views than others. Nevertheless, insensitivity to women in treatment can be highlighted by the lack of basic facilities, such as crèches, women-only spaces or time-slots, and of the presence of more imaginative services, such as health screening and information services, focused on their needs.[1] Being sensitive to women in treatment settings may depend upon any number of other factors – access to financial resources; the presence of a flexible, far-sighted boss or leader; the treatment centre's location in the city, its physical setting, the structure and layout of the building; the level of commitment of staff; whether or not there are clear treatment policies around gender, race, able-bodiness and class issues, and so on. Perhaps the most distinguishing factor in women-sensitive treatment agencies is the ability to recognise that women's problems with alcohol are rooted in their common experiences as women; their difficulties in dealing with women's specific problems; and the 'million other underlying problems' that women are likely to have.[2] As one woman who experienced negative drinking for a number of years said:

> Women have a lot of difficulties admitting to their drink problems. Women are ashamed to admit it . . . Any

treatment centre that is worth its salt is going to address women's issues and problems. It needs to attract women who are hidden about their drinking and sometimes full of shame.

In this context it is useful to know that advertising an alcohol treatment agency as offering a 'special service for women' is very different from actually providing a service that is women-sensitive. One must always read between the lines. In other words, when an agency advertises that it recognises women's needs, it may not do so in practice. Indeed, when I carried out a survey on women's use of alcohol and drug services in London,[3] various treaters told me that they advertised their services as 'women-sensitive'. When I explored this issue further, I discovered that for these treaters 'women-sensitive' meant merely that at that moment their centres had 'women in attendance'.

Most if not all of these treatment centres or agencies had previously had a policy of admitting women to their treatment settings, but women only came forward to them for treatment in rare cases. Thus, at the time of my survey, when the issue of providing services for a growing number of women needing treatment was gaining prominence,[4] treaters equated 'women in attendance' at their centre with 'women-sensitivity', regardless of the fact that their treatment policies on women had not changed in the least.

Unfortunately, services that are women-sensitive in name only can be set up as a way of getting more government money, attracting more clients when numbers are low, or building a respectable image in the local community. If services for women are to be improved and become more women-sensitive, service providers may need to change their attitudes towards women (ie those based on gendered judgements) and, more important, be more open to ideas and treatment approaches, geared towards women's needs.[5] In the alcohol field, translating ideas for change into action is a complex social process, requiring gender-sensitive information, careful consideration and sensitive strategies to make women visible.[6]

Certain strategies can be useful when we want to assess what is actually happening for women in local alcohol treatment services. For example, as a result of my experience with the survey described above, I now ask service providers in treatment agencies probing, if not difficult, questions when I hear that they are offering special services for women. I ask questions to find out whether I myself would consider going there if I needed help or whether I would send a woman who needs help to that agency.

Usually I ask what this special service for women means on a day-to-day level. Here are examples of questions I may ask: Do 'special services for women' mean that women have more choices, fewer choices or no choices in what is offered to them? Are differences between women recognised? Are women's problems seen as different in relation to men's problems? Do treaters accept that women's problems may arise around their experiences of shame, secrecy, child care, domestic violence, poor self-esteem, sexual abuse, and so on? Are women allowed to choose from any number of special services or are certain treatment practices (ie attending a women's group) obligatory?[7]

If coercion is involved in the treatment process, this can mean that the services being offered are rather rigid and may not be geared to women's needs. Coercion in a treatment setting may be opposed to healing, especially for women. Pressure and coercion have been central in these women's lives and specifically when they have been overdrinking, they have often felt 'forced' to drink.[8]

In this context, not every woman may want to attend a

women-only group. Women may find one-to-one counselling, co-counselling in a mixed-sex setting, or private, family or couple therapy more comfortable options. It has also been suggested that women in treatment centres could 'alternate between single-sex and mixed-sex groups with special support groups for women'.[9] Women need to experience a sense of creativity and social agency as they go through the healing process,[10] and they fare better when treatments are voluntary rather than compulsory.[11]

Now, let us move beyond the traditional treatment setting into the area of self-help, the main focus of this chapter. First we will look at the self-help group, Alcoholics Anonymous, as it has developed over the years in the alcohol field. Then, we will examine the co-dependency movement. It is important to make these studies in order to find out what self-help means for women with alcohol problems.

ALCOHOLICS ANONYMOUS

Alcoholics Anonymous (AA) is one of the oldest and most established self-help groups in the world. AA was founded in 1935 in Akron, Ohio, by Bill Wilson and Dr Bob Smith, both 'alcoholics'.[12] AA offers a 12-step programme of recovery to alcoholics who want to stop drinking. In 1939, four years after its establishment, AA had around 50 members – all men. Today AA is still predominantly male focused, although there are now many female AA members.

If a woman is thinking of joining AA, she may want to remember that it is a male-initiated programme and check that her needs are likely to be met. Here, let us ask three questions: What are self-help groups? Where does AA fit into this picture? and How have women fared so far in AA?

What are self-help groups?

The idea of self-help is a complex one and has wider social implications than its dictionary definition: 'the act or an instance of providing for or helping oneself without dependence on others'. For example, there are many reasons for joining self-help groups and there are many forms of self-help. If we look at the history of self-help groups, we can divide self-help groups into two types: the clinical or traditional type (ie focusing on the 'deviant' individual) and the structural or non-traditional type (ie focusing on the group of members who challenge society's views of deviants).[13]

Within the clinical type of group, self-help is seen as a desirable way of dealing with one's problems in small groups where one is expected to disclose something personal, perhaps painful, about oneself. Usually, people join these groups because they want to learn how to survive in a world from which they have been excluded because of their problems. For example, one overeats, overdrinks, has a sibling who is a drug addict, feels addicted to sex, and so on. Somehow, these people see themselves as not ideally suited for society.

In the structural type of group, self-help is seen as a natural process or an appropriate way to organise for people concerned about some change either in themselves or society. People tend to join these groups because they want to generate social awareness. For example, they discover that the city council is planning to put a motorway through their back gardens. So they start a local group to protest against these plans. They discover growing racism directed towards ethnic minorities in their local community. They start a local group to plan ways of tackling racism. In each example, people organise in local neighbourhoods for personal and social satisfaction and because they want to change what is going on around them.

Taking a closer look at these two types of self-help groups shows that individuals belonging to clinical groups may struggle to survive in a world in which they may not be ideally suited. Individual education rather than the consciousness of the group is seen as a way of changing things – whether it be their (ie group members') lives, attitudes, ideas or behaviour. In this way, people in clinical groups do not focus on changing society or its attitudes. Society has stigmatised them, and they will educate themselves on how best to live with that stigma.

On the other hand, members of structural self-help groups tend to reject social labels and stigmas. Their aim is to create a collective awareness of local and/or social problems and somehow to generate social change. Group consciousness takes priority over education, while members emphasise their basic human rights. These types of groups tend to question why society does not provide more resources for the kinds of issues they are engaged in.

Where does AA fit into this picture?

On a world scale, AA is probably the most well-known, socially acceptable self-help group for men and women 'alcoholics'. In some ways, AA fits into the above ideas on traditional self-help groups.[14] Men and women join AA because they want to stop drinking. They want to be able to survive in a society in which they have been labelled and stigmatised as 'drunks'. People with drinking problems may feel that they should turn to AA because traditional forms of alcohol treatment have failed them. However, people don't usually join AA because they feel like 'treatment failures'. Men and women who have never stepped foot through the door of a treatment agency find AA very helpful.

Because of their sometimes overwhelming problems with alcohol intake, members of AA find that their behaviour does not correspond very well with others in 'outside society'. In this context, AA can be seen to provide a needed shelter for its members.

All AA members follow the AA way of life, which is based on the already famous 12-step-programme.[15] For AA members, saying the words 'I am an alcoholic' usually means that they accept this 'alcoholic' label as a permanent fixture in their lives. In other words, 'Once an alcoholic always an alcoholic.' The assumptions behind the alcoholic definition used in AA tend to uphold a disease view of alcoholism – those who overdrink are sick. Regardless of that fact, members admit that they were powerless over alcohol and many learn to take personal responsibility for their lives. The anonymous nature of AA distances members from any form of political action, and AA is not a self-help group for social change. Nevertheless, over the years AA has helped vast numbers of people face their problems with drinking, and many have experienced personal transformation. The worth of AA for these people must be neither denied nor underestimated. One woman member who found AA helpful to her says:

> AA is a good way of getting your act together and getting your show on the road.

However, although in recent years AA has offered women's groups, the predominantly mixed settings (ie with both men and women present) of AA meetings has not always been an ideal setting for women. Add to that setting different age groups, races, sexual orientations, able-bodiness, social classes and ethnic origins, we find a microcosm of society. How does AA deal with social inequalities amongst its members? From women members' points of view, how does AA deal with the inequality of gender?

How have women fared so far in AA?

Another way of asking this last question would be: How have women fared so far in AA? In order to find an answer, we need to focus on one of the first women to join AA: Marty Mann. Marty became quite famous internationally in the alcohol field and she founded the National Council on Alcoholism in the USA. From 1969 until 1980, the year of her death, she sponsored[16] a woman named Jane. In an interview with Sarah Hafner,[17] Jane talks about Marty Mann's life. Through Jane's words, we see that becoming a member of AA was not easy for Marty because 'women were not expected to become alcoholics'. Jane talked about Marty's first AA meeting.

During the early years of AA, weekly Tuesday evening meetings were held at the house of one of the founders, Bill Wilson, in Brooklyn Heights, New York. There were no women. Jane remembers Marty's words:

'Bill's house was on a nice quite street. As soon as we were in Brooklyn Heights, as soon as we entered, I knew, I just knew, I couldn't go in there. That had been the trouble all along. All my life I had needed a drink in order to meet new people. How could I possibly do something as important as this without a drink?' So she fled to the bedroom where the coats were being kept and flung herself on top of them weeping. Eventually a woman came in and sat down beside her and placed her hand gently on Marty's shoulder and she said, 'Please come in. We've been waiting for you for a very, very long time.' Of course this woman was Lois, Bill's wife. She herself was not an alcoholic, but had lived with Bill's alcoholism for so long, she became as much a sponsor to Marty as Bill was. She was the only woman for [Marty] to talk to for the longest while.[18]

When Marty Mann became the first woman member of AA, the male members were astonished because they thought she was a freak.[19] In the early years, women could not be active AA members.[20] Women were present only within the confines of Al-Anon, a group set up initially for wives of alcoholics. But gradually this changed as some women, like Marty Mann, gained a vital presence within AA.

Jane continues to speak for Marty:

> The men in the group felt that there was no such thing as a woman alcoholic. They were, in other words, an exception to the rule. They were not saying a woman could not be an alcoholic, just that they were real oddities.[21]

Women are now active members within AA. However, it was difficult in the early days for women alcoholics to challenge the idea, held by male members, that they were 'real oddities'. This absence of women in the early days of AA should not be surprising, given that AA began as a 'fellowship', a term which suggests a gendered interest. The traditional focus of AA has been on the male breadwinner as the head of the family and restoring 'his' family to normal. The world-famous *The AA Way of Life: A Reader by Bill* (Wilson, one of AA's founders) makes this point clear:

> Though an alcoholic does not respond, there is no reason why you should neglect his [sic] family. You should continue to be friendly to them, explaining AA's concept of alcoholism and its treatment. If they accept this and also apply our principles to their problems, there is a better chance that the head of the family will recover.[22]

In this same discussion, Bill emphasises that a related but separate self-help group, Al-Anon, has been established for families and that the initiation of the AA way of life in the home is the central purpose of Al-Anon family groups.[23] Since 1967 when the *Reader* was published, members of AA have made little if any attempt to question the centrality of men's position within the family.

One woman member of AA spoke with me at great length about other women members she had encountered. Below, she gives her views as well as an account of her own experiences in AA and in AA women's groups. She believes that the male focus of AA does unavoidably influence women members. She points out that in some ways, women may be made to feel inferior, voiceless, uncomfortable and even left out. She believes it is often easier for a man than a woman to go to AA meetings:

> . . . Because he is a man, he is OK. Yes, he has got problems but at least he is one of the boys . . . When he goes to an AA meeting, there are lots of men there. He makes a lot of friends and becomes one of the boys in the fellowship. Women find it extremely difficult.

The picture painted by this woman was not, however, totally pessimistic. She offers a more hopeful picture when she reflects on changes that she has witnessed over 20 years of membership. For her, some women are able to speak and communicate more now than in the past. She saw this as a 'generational change'. In other words, more younger women and professional women were becoming members and they appeared to be more confident in speaking out in male-dominated settings. But she noted that in spite of changes in AA's female constituency, there are visible and enormous differences amongst the women. In her view, some women, of all ages, still do not feel comfortable disclosing anything about themselves — let alone telling their life stories, as is required of members.

For some women attending mixed meetings may prove to

be a difficult as well as painful experience. In this woman's view, the experiences of female members are coloured by both what some male members say and how they say it. In the end, some women may be 'horrified' if male members' ways of expressing their masculinity are intimidatory. She continues:

> A lot of women are not going to walk into a room and all of a sudden be able to be immediately absorbed by the group. First, they might be horrified listening to all of the macho stories . . .

So, the often masculine style of AA meetings and the sometimes excessively masculine (ie 'macho') stories may serve to block the healing process for some women. For that reason, this woman felt that women's groups rather than mixed groups within AA were extremely helpful and necessary. She also believes that women's groups help not only to bring women out of their 'isolation' but also to address their problems in a particular way, even if this means that a woman goes into treatment. She continues:

> The women's groups serve a very useful function in getting women together and putting them out of their isolation. Maybe they go over the top and embarrass their husbands. As a result, they do not go out. This is a vicious circle situation. So they join a women's group. But, even so, some of these women go into treatment. This is because it may be the only way they can address their problems. This is a relevant point.

So AA women's groups help some women to open up and face their problems. These groups also provide a type of non-threatening atmosphere which gives women the power to speak. This woman also described how the experience of hearing other women's stories gives women permission to talk about themselves:

> Whenever I hear that one particular woman is in the chair and speaking, I go to these AA women's meetings. Time and again I go to hear her story. It is an experience. She says my name is [name of woman] and she begins by crying. Then she says, 'I am an alcoholic'. I feel that as she cries and the tears come, we get this riveting story. Of course, there is not a dry eye in the house. But, you see, this sort of experience gives women permission to do the same sort of thing . . . For a lot of women they need to hear and to see this.

From the above words, we see that AA originated primarily as a group for male alcoholics, but that it has changed over the years to include female alcoholics. However, not all women approaching AA today may find their needs met within the 'AA fellowship'. Jean Kirkpatrick, for example, founded Women for Sobriety in 1978 because she believed that 'the AA programme does not meet the needs of everyone, especially not women'.[24] For her, AA was overly identified with male problems, regardless of the development of women-only groups within AA. Jean Kirkpatrick believes that Women for Sobriety provides a more favourable space for women's healing process. While AA focuses on individual, personal disclosure of intimate secrets and life stories (which women may find a disempowering process), Women for Sobriety provides space for women 'to take charge of themselves'.[25]

Rather than confessing intimate personal details, which can be, for women alcoholics, surrounded with emotions such as shame and self-disgust, a more positive technique might be consciousness-raising.[26] Consciousness-raising involves discussing and learning more about factors in society that lead to the problems women experience. It therefore rejects blaming women for their problems. Consciousness-raising is a powerful dynamic of healing. It also stresses the common issues women face and leads to expressions of empathy and understanding within the group. Through consciousness-raising, women may find that there are other women who share their destructive experiences with alcohol. In consciousness-raising groups, a sense of reciprocity through sharing is able to develop and members are able to experience what it means to be equal in a group of alcoholics because consciousness-raising is non-hierarchical. Although these women may recognise differences amongst each other, women may also find that these differences fade when they are giving or receiving empathic responses with other women. Consciousness-raising helps to foster female friendships. As suggested in the previous chapter, women tend to heal themselves in friendship and thus consciousness-raising, by giving rise to and then emphasising the strength of female friendships, can aid women-healing.

While women's groups have become an established part of AA, some women may want to explore other self-help possibilities besides AA. They may want to join Women for Sobriety, for example, or set up their own self-help groups. Others may want to become active in the co-dependency movement. Whatever creative steps women take, they need courage and they need to do whatever is necessary to gain strength and healing in their lives.

THE CO-DEPENDENCY MOVEMENT

Alongside the rise of AA, the growth of its 'relative', the co-dependency movement, has been witnessed in recent years. In looking at the issue of self-help with gender-sensitive eyes, an exploration of co-dependency is helpful. At the beginning of this chapter, it was stated that studying what makes women strong should allow women to make more choices for themselves but, more importantly, to know what these choices are. Becoming active in the co-dependency movement may be a woman's choice, but she needs to choose with open eyes.

The idea of co-dependency has gained much currency in the alcohol field since the publication in 1986 of an influential book, *Co-dependence: misunderstood – mistreated.*[27] At heart, these ideas are based on the view that family members or those living in a close relationship with an alcoholic organise their lives around an alcoholic's conduct. This means that these 'significant others' themselves are part of the disease process. For example, wives, spouses or children are viewed and very often view themselves as 'co-alcoholics' or 'co-dependents'.

One professional women, Jane Sloven, who works in this area describes the force of co-dependency:

> This process allowed everyone in the family to have a 'disease' from which they could 'recover'. The twelve steps of AA and Al-Anon could then be utilised by 'co-dependents' as a way of learning to live their own lives, regardless of the behaviour of the chemically dependent person. As children of alcoholics began to receive attention and treatment, and adult children of alcoholics began to identify the consequences of growing up in alcoholic families, the concept of codependency grew.[28]

Of course, there are many variations on the co-dependency theme. The idea of co-dependency has been applied to all sorts of substances and abusive relationships. Co-dependency has been used in official treatment settings as well as within self-help groups such as Adult Children of Alcoholics or Co-dependents Anonymous. This idea, co-dependency, offers an apparently neat package in the form of the dysfunctional, diseased family or the abusive, addictive relationship. But this co-dependency package is not so neat. In fact, hidden within this movement is a tendency to stigmatise women. This is because those speaking so eloquently about co-dependency may, albeit unconsciously, put somewhat negative images or damaging labels on women, who in their view, are co-dependent. As a result, women once again become the targets of harmful labels and destructive views. This targeting may make it impossible for them to heal their wounds in peace.

Let us study the above ideas more closely and ask, 'What really happens to women, particularly wives or partners of male alcoholics, in this co-dependency movement?' If a woman is involved with an alcoholic man,[29] she is told that she is afflicted with a disease – the disease of relating to an alcoholic. In order to fully recover, she along with her partner needs to accept a victim role – both she and her male partner are diseased. There is not much she can do about this, only accept it. As the co-alcoholic, she is addicted to, dependent upon, hooked to, etc her 'alcoholic', abusive relationship. This is regardless of the fact that she may have never put á glass of alcohol to her lips. This fact is somehow immaterial – she too is hooked. Therefore, she needs treatment. Someone needs to do something to change her. This someone may also need to take a large sum of money from her, if she decides to go into treatment as a 'co-alcoholic'/'co-dependent'.

The label 'co-dependent' may not be as healing as it appears to be, especially for women. It is possible that women are being punished, stigmatised, and victimised when they are labelled 'co-dependent'. The main reason for treating 'co-dependent' women in this way is because they appear to be caring. Maybe, they have been a little over-responsible or over-protective of their partners or themselves. Perhaps, they have cared a little too much. This is what some women who have been in the co-dependency movement have said:

> After all, I have remained in the relationship, however painful or destructive it has been for me. Love and caring [are] not always easy. You have to take the good with the bad.

or

> Anyway, I was afraid to leave [partner]. I felt responsible to stay.

or

> I was ashamed to walk out that door. How could I abandon [partner] in a time of need?

or

> What about the children? – What would happen to them? – They could be put into care, you know.

or

> How would I have survived on my own? If [partner] left, who would pay the mortgage? – on my salary – forget it!

On the one hand, these 'co-dependent' women have been aware of society's rules. These rules of feminine behaviour have been ingrained in them from a very early age. As a result, they may also be aware of hidden social messages to women: 'You must please others', 'You must be nice', 'You must care for others', 'You must be nurturing', 'You must be responsible in relationships', 'You must keep the family together', etc. Indeed, women have played by these rules and heard these messages sometimes at a great cost to themselves – to their careers, their health, their emotional life, and so on.

On the other hand, 'co-dependent' women are being blamed for playing by society's rules. An accusing finger is pointed at them. Inside themselves a voice may be saying, 'But I am supposed to care for my partner, surely?' Here one could ask, 'What are women supposed to do in these circumstances?' In the co-dependency view, women are informed that they are afflicted with the disease of relating to an alcoholic. This is regardless of the fact that these women may be making healthy psychological attempts to salvage their damaged relationships. It may be difficult for them to see anything wrong with themselves and given that they wholeheartedly embrace their caring and nurturing roles.

One unmarried heterosexual woman who is currently dating a man she plans to marry has been active in the co-dependency movement. She had been involved in a self-help group for co-dependents in her local community for about a year. She talks about her experience:

> All of us in my group have found out that we have been tightly bound to abusive relationships all of our lives – in the family and outside our families. What we learn in the family we just carry over into our other relationships. We need to learn about the addiction of our relationships – how these relationships give a compulsive touch to our lives. We need to learn independence.

In my view, the idea of co-dependency confirms a traditional view: the centrality of relationships in women's lives and women's almost total responsibility for maintaining relationships. Also, the idea of co-dependency leaves unanswered questions around the construction of power and the process of healing in these relationships. For example, a woman is told that she is abnormal and affected by a partner's behaviour – she is diseased like an alcoholic and thus labelled 'co-alcoholic'. While her 'co-alcoholism' may have something to do with her partner's (ie the person who actually has the alcohol problem) abusive behaviour, it is also in her.

'Co-alcoholism' becomes her problem by the fact that she got involved in this 'alcoholic' relationship. For example, although a woman may try very hard to understand her partner's problem and give support, she appears to have been drawn into this relationship like someone drawn to alcohol. It is almost as if the relationship becomes an addictive 'cocktail'. In the end, women are blamed for pursuing this 'alcoholic' relationship. This picture presents a somewhat distorted view of the reality of these women's lives. The co-dependency movement tends to ignore the complexities of women's problems, emerging on many levels.[30] Here, I mention three examples of the complexities of women's problems – to do with levels of dependency, problem solving and hurt – in order to show how the co-dependency movement distorts women's situations.

The level of dependency

It is quite normal to be touched by those with whom one has a primary relationship and to be affected by their behaviour. For whatever reasons (eg because we love them, we are afraid to be alone, they are the only ones who understand us, we have good times together, we still have sex together after 16 years, we have three beautiful children, we have a lovely house, and so on), a woman may feel quite dependent upon her partner. She needs him or her. There is such a thing as basic, human dependency. We need each other and depend upon each other. This is regardless of who has the most power in the relationship, what others outside of the relationship may say, and whether or not others see this type of dependency as healthy. 'Co-dependency' tends to ignore this level of reality.

The level of problem solving

If 'co-alcoholism' is a woman's problem and not her partner's, how is this problem to be solved? Her partner is also involved in this relationship. Does he or she share some responsibility for solving problems within this relationship? For example, one woman says:

> I have been stigmatised for being 'other focused', focusing on you and your problems. Now you and the experts see our relationship as my problem. Why? If I feel hurt in my relationship to you, I am unable to heal myself by merely being independent from you. I am not going to be strong by simply disconnecting. In order to heal, I need to heal in the relationship, regardless of what may happen in the future. If possible, we need to remember or even to find the hidden, perhaps long-gone friendship on which our relationship was presumably once based. We need to take mutual responsibility for what happens between us. I refuse to be blamed for your alcohol problem or to take responsibility for your behaviour.

This level of problem solving tends to be skewed through ideas of 'co-dependency'.

The level of hurt

If a 'co-dependent' woman has been emotionally or physically hurt because of her partner's alcohol problem, she can be viewed as the primary cause of her own hurt. Of course, if physical violence, sexual abuse or rape is involved, her sensations of hurt may alter greatly. To experience these kinds of hurt against her will in an 'alcoholic' relationship is not about her being involved in a disease process. That view is a distortion because these kinds of hurt are purely and simply male violence against a woman. In this situation, a woman may say:

> It is your mouth that has spewed the cruel, vicious words, while your powerful fists have struck the hurtful blows to my face and body. The experts and you yourself may call me co-dependent, co-alcoholic, but I see myself as your normal, average female partner of an alcoholic male who is violent. If you want to label me, wounded woman will suffice.

Because of its individualistic focus, the co-dependency view does not offer a clear picture of violence against women.

BECOMING STRONG

In an attempt to move towards an appreciation of women-healing, this chapter has studied a variety of areas. We have looked at the importance of women-sensitive services in treatment and we have reviewed self-help ideas in AA and the co-dependency movement. The aim has been to see some of the choices for healing available to women in the alcohol field. However, as we have seen, these choices are limited.

Nevertheless, it was suggested earlier that women need to learn to help themselves to do that which gives them strength. Therefore, women need to avoid situations in which they know that they will end up feeling bad about themselves, in which they become labelled as victims or where they are forced to accept a victim role. Women need to avoid and possibly reject people who make them feel inferior, shameful, not good enough or unworthy of help and human compassion. Simply, in helping herself, a woman must ensure that she avoids further harm and woundings.

Taking this creative, healing step may not be easy for some women. This is because more often than not women's lives as well as the processes of helping and healing one's female self have been controlled by others. A woman's bodily and emotional hungers may have been governed by a bottle – one full of alcohol. For any woman to take control of her life, her body, her health and her problems with alcohol is a radical, creative step. It is to develop a strong sense of her female self – an empowering experience.

In this context, as suggested earlier, women are starved of images of strong women that are women defined. More often than not women are afraid of their own female strength. This strength is viewed as selfish and destructive because it challenges women's images of themselves as carers and as other-focused. It is hard for many women to think of themselves without thinking that they are somehow egocentric, egotistic, self-centred or self-indulgent.

However, we can be hopeful because one of the labels I have mentioned could be very empowering: that is the label of wounded woman. This suggests that a woman can have been harmed by something that is not her fault and that she has a right to healing and care. It also suggests the wider circumstances of being a woman – that women in general are often vulnerable to wounding because of the society in which they live. Many wounded women have had the experience that their greatest strength is their vulnerability. Vulnerability involves sensing our own pain or wounded feelings, and many women find that owning their feelings helps them to own their power.[31] In other words, once we know what makes us vulnerable, what gives us pain and wounds us, we can start to face it. Once we face it, we can start to find ways to deal with it. And then we begin to sense our own power. So, when wounded women allow themselves to feel their vulnerability, they experience, at the same time, feelings of strength, power, and a sense of human purpose. While someone may take away these women's alcohol bottles, with the result that they feel lonely and hopeless, no one can take away the strength that comes from owning and feeling their vulnerability.

That the experience of vulnerability can be one's strength is perhaps a difficult notion to comprehend. This idea suggests what Nor Hall[32] calls an 'alchemical' truth and is, therefore, about transforming something common – vulnerability – into something precious – strength. Related to this idea, Nor Hall suggests that 'the cure of an emotional wound is in the wound itself'.[33]

There are few well-defined images or models of strong women for wounded women to follow. Some women may have a tendency to be afraid of their own strength; to view this strength as potentially destructive; or to feel ashamed, selfish and self-centred when they feel strong. The notion that vulnerability is our strength brings us inevitably back to ourselves – our inner female selves. To heal this inner female self is to enter into our wounds and to dip into our scars. While this may be a frightening experience, full of anguish, we may find an unimaginable power and vitality unleashed in this healing process.

Notes

1.   See Jan Waterson and Betsy Ettorre, 'Providing Services for Women with Difficulties with Alcohol and Other Drugs: The Current UK Situation as Seen by Women Practitioners, Researchers and Policy Makers in the Field', *Drug and Alcohol Dependence* 24 (1989): 119–25. In this context, we found that major shortcomings in the treatment field included a lack of special facilities for women,

theoretical understanding of how women's problems started, and information and training on women's special needs.

2. In Bridgid McConville, *Women Under the Influence: Alcohol and its Impact* (New York: Schocken Books, 1983), pp 132–34, a social worker describes in detail how women's problems with alcohol are linked closely to their experiences as women generally.

3. See Drugs Alcohol and Women Nationally (DAWN), with assistance from Dr EM Ettorre, *A Survey of Facilities for Women Using Drugs (Including Alcohol)* (London: DAWN, 1985).

4. Betsy Thom, 'Women and Alcohol: The Emergence of a Risk Group', in Maryon McDonald, ed, *Gender, Drink and Drugs* (Oxford: Berg, 1994). See especially the sections 'The changing face of alcoholism: from the female alcoholic to women's drinking' and 'Policy responses to women's drinking' on pp 43–46 and 46–49, respectively.

5. Jan Waterson and Betsy Ettorre, 'Providing Services for Women with Difficulties with Alcohol or Drug Problems: The Current UK Situation as Seen by Women Practitioners, Researchers and Policy Makers in the Field', p 124.

6. Bam Bjorling, 'Making Women Visible', in Elina Haavio-Mannila, ed, *Women, Alcohol and Drugs in the Nordic Countries* (Helsinki: Nordic Council for Alcohol and Drug Research, 1989).

7. Jean Shinoda Bolen notes how important it is for women with alcohol problems to learn how to become what she calls 'choicemakers' and that this process must be done 'gradually', without force. See Bolen, *Goddesses in Everywoman: A New Psychology of Women* (New York: Harper and Row Publishers, 1985), p 293.

8. In Bridgid McConville's discussions with treaters, it became clear that a lot of women who overdrink are often under a lot of pressure in their domestic situations. At times, these women don't have any other choice than to relieve their depressive feelings by drinking. See *Women Under the Influence*, pp 126–30.

9. Fanny Duckert, 'The Treatment of Female Problem Drinkers', in Elina Haavio-Mannila, ed, *Women, Alcohol and Drugs in the Nordic Countries*, p 182.

10. Elizabeth Ettorre, 'Substance Use and Women's Health', in Sue Wilkinson and Celia Kitzinger, eds, *Women and Health: Feminist Perspectives* (London: Taylor and Francis, 1994).

11. It is important here to emphasise that treatment settings must somehow obtain a delicate balance between giving support, offering

healing or providing a safe container for women, and being flexible and open-minded. A woman client must be prepared to be aware of her rights and responsibilities in getting treatment. She must be aware that she may need to take certain risks in order to heal. See the chapter 'Outside help' in Rosemary Kent, *Say When!: Everything a Woman Needs to Know about Alcohol and Drinking Problems* (London: Sheldon Press, 1990), pp 79–90.

12. Alcoholics Anonymous, *Twelve Steps and Twelve Traditions* (Aylesbury, UK: Hazell, Watson and Viney Ltd, 1974, seventh British printing).

13. This typology can be found in DL Pancoast, P Parker and C Froland, eds, *Rediscovering Self-Help: Its Role in Social Care* (Beverly Hills, CA: Sage Publications, 1983). Also, I have used these types as models in describing the emergence of tranquilliser self-help groups. See EM Ettorre, 'Self-Help Groups as an Alternative to Benzodiazepine Use'. in Jonathan Gabe and Paul Williams, eds, *Tranquillisers: Social, Psychological and Clinical Perspectives* (London: Tavistock. 1986).

14. There is also Al-Anon for relatives of alcoholics and Al-Ateen for teenagers. More recent groups have been Women for Sobriety and CODA (Co-Dependents Anonymous). We will discuss the co-dependency movement later in this chapter.

15. Alcoholics Anonymous, *The AA Way of Life: A Reader by Bill* (London: AA Publishing Company, 1967).

16. AA has a system of sponsorship amongst its members. Every member has a sponsor, guiding them through the 12 steps and recovery. One's sponsor may also act as a type of personal counsellor when one is in need or crisis.

17. See the very interesting book by Sarah Hafner, *Nice Girls Don't Drink: Stories of Recovery* (New York: Bergin and Garvey, 1992) for accounts of 'recovering women alcoholics'. The following account of Marty Mann by Jane is taken from this book.

18. Sarah Hafner, *Nice Girls Don't Drink*, pp 223–24.

19. Sarah Hafner, *Nice Girls Don't Drink*, pp 223–24.

20. See, for example, Alcoholics Anonymous, *The Story of How Many Thousands of Men and Women Have Recovered from Alcoholism* (Aylesbury, UK: Hazell, Watson and Viney Ltd, 1963). The emphasis in this book is on men, although this point is raised in Chapter 8, 'To wives', p 117.

21. Sarah Hafner, *Nice Girls Don't Drink*, pp 223–24.

22. Alcoholics Anonymous, *The AA Way of Life: A Reader by Bill*, p 190.

23. Alcoholics Anonymous, *The AA Way of Life: A Reader by Bill*, p 190.

24. Jean Kirkpatrick, 'Preface', *Turnabout: New Help for the Woman Alcoholic* (Seattle: Madrona Publishers, 1986), p 1.

25. Jean Kirkpatrick, 'Preface', *Turnabout*, p 1.

26. Consciousness-raising (CR) originated from small groups of women within the women's movement who wanted to focus on their individual and collective experiences and change their lives with the support of other women. A 'classic' article on the dynamics of CR is Kathie Sarachild, 'Consciousness Raising: A Radical Weapon', in Kathie Sarachild, ed, *Feminist Revolution* (New York: Radstockings, 1975).

27. See AW Schaef, *Co-dependence: Misunderstood – Mistreated* (Minneapolis: Winston Press, 1986).

28. See Jane Sloven, 'Codependent or Empathically Responsive?: Two Views of Betty', in Claudia Bepko, ed, *Feminism and Addiction* (New York, London and Sydney: The Haworth Press, 1991), for an excellent discussion on this topic.

29. Here, I should emphasise that this 'alcoholic partner' can also be a woman. For example, a 'co-dependent relationship' may also refer to a lesbian relationship in which one of the partners is 'alcoholic' and the other is 'co-alcoholic'. In this context, I am referring to male/female heterosexual relationships.

30. The powerful writing of Jane Sloven in this area is inspiring. Many of the ideas which I discuss concerning the levels where women's problems arise were originally hers. Another piece of writing has also been influential here: M Mason's 'Women and Shame: Kin and Culture', also in Claudia Bepko, ed, *Feminism and Addiction*.

31. Sheila Ernst and Lucy Goodison, *In Our Own Hands: A Book of Self-Help Therapy* (London: The Women's Press, 1981), p 19.

32. See Nor Hall, *The Moon and the Virgin* (London: The Women's Press, 1980), especially pp 68–69.

33. Nor Hall, *The Moon and the Virgin*, pp 68–69.

CHAPTER 6

Mixing women-sensitivity with alcohol: a Molotov cocktail?

INTRODUCTION

In an attempt to look towards the future, I will, in this final chapter, focus first on strategies for change and then on new approaches to theory. In the context of this book, the ideas presented in this chapter are aimed at providing the final touches to a comprehensive picture on the issue of women and alcohol. As we all know, having good ideas is not the same as putting these ideas into practice. When a woman is an overdrinker, she not only needs to know that she has constructive ideas about changing her life, but also that she has the power to put these ideas into practice effectively.

Overdrinking women need clear ways of challenging the negative attitudes that exist about them. But, as implied throughout the previous discussions, to produce these strategies is not an easy task, and women need to sense their needs in the context of a social group of others who are overdrinkers. Membership of this group is all about gathering strength and courage through a deep recognition of one's vulnerability. We explore, in this chapter, how women can develop a sense of collective needs and learn strategic actions through shared visions.

SEEING WOMEN

So far in our discussions, we have seen that generally those who have studied alcohol have been resistant to the needs of women. Often, the wider social implications of being a woman, the differences between men and women and the gendering of their relations have been ignored. In this light, underlying questions throughout this book have been: How can women's experiences with alcohol, whether negative or not, be recognised and valued? and How can a women-sensitive perspective develop? The 'herstories' hidden within discussions on women and alcohol have been uncovered by asking these questions. In effect, the women and alcohol issue has been placed alongside critical ideas on gender, and a well-established area of study has been looked at in a different light.

Given the pace of life in the world today, it is fair to say that most if not all people live both their public and private lives surrounded by stress. On a public level, one sees and experiences a sense of social and even global stress. Rapid social changes; threats to our planet's environment, whether through possible nuclear extinction or uncontrollable pollution; rising unemployment in 'developed' countries; growing poverty, famine and disease in 'developing' countries; and inter-regional conflicts and wars exist. On a private level, one may experience psychological stress through depression, anxiety, family breakdown, sickness and a general sense of malaise. All of us live with stress. Stress has become a major feature of modern society, and it is experienced by various individuals, social groups and societies in different degrees of intensity.

With this experience of living in stress, many women take on all the requirements of being a 'proper female' or a good woman in society. Soon they find, however, that because of this stress their emotional lives and psychological or physical well-being are in jeopardy. While women use most health services more often than men,[1] women may find that their dependence on substances, whether or not these are addictive, becomes an important way of dealing with stress. In a real sense, they can no longer be depended upon in the traditional ways society expects women care givers to behave.

Within the field of alcohol, a sensitivity to these issues remains hidden. In the final analysis, this level of sensitivity is not valued. Here, the genealogy of women's collective struggle and survival with alcohol as a potentially addictive substance should be outlined. Simply, there is a continual need to examine women's experiences with alcohol and to recognise that these experiences reflect the constant struggle for women to maintain their integrity and self-worth in a substance-using, anxiety-ridden society that does not value women.

CREATING VISIONS

What are we able to say about the future for women alcohol users both as individuals and as a group? Sharing visions may help to build a picture of what personal and broader types of change can mean to those who want to gain strength and heal themselves as women overdrinkers. Creating visions can be a very rich and at times painful experience. It can be a rich experience because we see much potential in our changing lives, and it can be painful because we see how all of our struggles demand healing at some level.

To create a strong vision we need to develop a sense of our inner selves. Simply, in order to visualise possibilities for ourselves, we may need to become sensitive to ourselves as women at the core of our being – to get to know exactly what we need. This means that women need to direct their energies towards putting themselves and their needs first – something that can be very difficult for women, as we have to 'unlearn' our socialisation to put others first. This is a delicate, woman-oriented process – the distinct process whereby a woman searches to find what she really needs. Any woman who has suffered the pain of overdrinking may need to look deep inside herself to discover this.

This process can be likened to the search for the woman-in-me,[2] in which women learn to nurture or care for things unseen inside themselves. Some women, in moving away from their dependence on alcohol, find simultaneously a new independence in themselves. But it is not an easy process. It may be difficult for a woman to feel really free, independent and creative because her grief, sorrow, anger or frustration tends to pull her down. Often a woman's desire to speak as a vulnerable woman becomes swallowed up by doubts, hesitancies or ambivalences. On the other hand, another woman may feel mostly powerful and strong, with a positive vision of her future, but she may at times swing between feelings of power and powerlessness. For all such women, speaking out about the difficult issue of drinking can be very painful. One author describes the tension between feelings of power and powerlessness as a type of dance, specific to the experiences of wounded women: they become dancers who suffer as they speak.[3]

With these tensions, doubts and fears, however, creating visions may be a survival mechanism for many women. Visions give hope, but hope may not be enough. Women also need to link their visions and ideas about their lives, struggles and futures with actions in their everyday lives.

To create a sense of vision and develop strategic actions for women overdrinkers, let us ask two questions: How do we develop a sensitivity towards ourselves as women? and What strategies can be helpful to women overdrinkers in being more aware of their inner selves?

WHAT IS WOMEN-SENSITIVITY?

Another way of asking this question could be: 'What is the central ethic or main operating principle as women develop strategies for themselves?' First, any woman's creativity, healing and strength develop from an awareness of being a woman collectively with other women. What are the common factors in our situation? How can we work to overcome any problems that arise out of these? How can I nurture myself as a women? With such questions, we give ourselves primacy and importance. We put our needs first and resist putting others' needs before our own. We develop a sense of feeling powerful and concentrate our energy on our creativity as women. Then, we can work to develop self-confidence, a sense of inner strength, autonomy, clear thinking, assertiveness – all needed to move the boundaries within which we have traditionally had to operate.

To develop strategies for action, women need to excavate the variety of ways they use alcohol. They will need to challenge traditional ideas developed in a field where most, if not all, professionals and 'experts' are men.[4] As we have seen, women who experience problem drinking have been viewed as being sick, out of control, morally reprehensible and so on, and as a result, the integrity of women has been compromised. Labels have been slapped on them. But these labels have prevented people from looking beyond women's drinking to the broader realities of their lives. The strategy of looking beyond female labels to a full view of one's day-to-day life is essential if healing is to take place.

But labels are a somewhat easy way to put people into

boxes in society. Labels help those with power to make divisions between good and bad, strong and vulnerable, insiders and outsiders and what is seen as morally right and wrong. And to overcome the labels that are slapped on 'deviant' women such as alcoholics, women need to nurture their deepest selves.

WHAT STRATEGIES CAN BE HELPFUL TO WOMEN OVERDRINKERS IN BEING MORE AWARE OF THEIR INNER SELVES?

Susan Griffin[5] has said that when women learn to trust our own visions, we begin a transformative process. Women begin to build a conscious vessel, a container within themselves, a receptive inner self which challenges the uncertain, ambivalent and masculine fear of the feminine, which leads to ill-treatment or undervaluation of women in society. When we identify our common situation as women, we can start to overcome a view of ourselves as polluted, deviant, outcasts or non-women by the very fact that we are overdrinkers.

Let us look briefly at two key strategies which could help to preserve a positive sense of ourselves: first, becoming active in healing and second, making ourselves powerful to bring about change.

Becoming active in healing

Women need to know that it is not enough to move themselves away from pain, danger or hurtful situations. Women must move towards pleasure, action and positive ways of defining themselves. Most of all this is a healing process. Within it a woman is able to reaffirm her identity as a woman and to reject wholeheartedly negative labels such as 'drunken slut' or 'evil woman'.

Making a positive choice to heal oneself means that a woman accepts the many reasons why she has experienced negative drinking. She sees her choice to understand herself as creative and empowering. Simply, she sees that her overdrinking has been, at times, a chosen course of action in unpleasant, if not humiliating, situations. She does not excuse her destructiveness. Rather she sees it for what it is – a response to circumstances which are harming her. In this way, a woman becomes active in her own rehabilitation. She unleashes healing energy in a dynamic way.

Making ourselves powerful to bring about change

Many women are aware that they are not particularly powerful in society. But an awareness of this can be strengthening, not weakening. Many women accept that they are not and perhaps don't want to be powerful in a 'masculinist' sense (ie in the ways we have traditionally expected men to be). Some women may in fact dislike authoritarian structures. This dislike may be a form of resistance in which women are able to heal their wounds and strengthen their spirits. They may, for example, be highly aware that it is not a failing in them that they do not feel powerful or indeed have power, and they may feel strong in their lack of respect for the power structures that do exist.

Some women recognise that they are in a position to challenge hierarchical structures of power – for example, they may stand up for themselves when they recognise that they are being treated or spoken to in a derogatory way simply because they are women. They may start to see parallels between their situation as a woman and the situation of other people who are undervalued in society on the grounds of class or race. This can be very energising and empowering.

When a woman who has experienced overdrinking adopts

this approach, she rejects the idea that her overdrinking is due to her own personal failing. She starts to take action to overcome the real, broader causes of problems such as alcoholism. While the very fact of being conscious of their vulnerability is empowering, women can move towards engagement with that which empowers women. They would benefit from this engagement because it would become a transformation process. By exposing the full realities of their dependency on alcohol as women, they can struggle against the view that women's addiction is an individual problem and make visible the idea that addiction is a social problem as well as a women's issue.

CHALLENGING TRADITIONAL VIEWS: MYTH, HEALING AND THE FEMALE BODY

One aim of this chapter is to offer a conceptual framework in which to place new ideas about the women and alcohol issue. Three books are useful in developing this knowledge and challenging traditional views.[6] The first two – Jan Bauer's *Alcoholism and Women: The Background and the Psychology*[7] and Jean Kirkpatrick's *Turnabout: New Help for the Woman Alcoholic*[8] – have been written specifically from within the alcohol field by women writers sensitive to women's particular problems in relation to alcohol. The third book, Susan Griffin's *Woman and Nature: The Roaring Inside Her*,[9] does not emerge specifically from the alcohol field but is helpful for broader ideas about current notions of women's bodies.

All of these previous works help to develop ideas on the women and alcohol issue with regard to myths, healing and the female body. For example, Jan Bauer's book is concerned with mythological images and symbols of women's drinking.

One sees how and why socially accepted myths can be used as a way almost to justify overdrinking. Bauer discusses the deep hidden meanings that alcohol has in women's lives. That these meanings are unearthed provides one with a deeper sense of women's suffering and their at times ambivalent relationship to alcohol.

Jean Kirkpatrick's book develops ideas on healing. How can feelings of self-worth, self-esteem and self-value in a self-help context be empowering for women? As we already know from an earlier discussion, Jean Kirkpatrick is a self-confessed alcoholic and founder of Women for Sobriety. In her work, she invites women 'alcoholics' to develop a sense of themselves as competent female human beings, but she sees this sense as being particularly difficult for them.

The third work, by Susan Griffin, guides one to consider the importance of the female body and offers a view of women rooted in the struggle for liberation. It provides a women-oriented framework and explores women's relationship to themselves, their bodies, human nature, spirit and matter. It is a study on how to become a woman of substance. For Susan Griffin, women's liberation is deeply connected to the female body and how it is suppressed and controlled. In this context, making a connection between one's body and how to become a woman of substance may be a key issue for those experiencing problems with alcohol.

All of the above works can have an impact on the direction of one's thinking about women and alcohol. They provide the tools to examine quite thoroughly three levels of experience: the mythological, healing and the bodily level. The assumption here is that all of these levels of experience can be problematic for women in their relationship to alcohol and intrude upon women's lives in unseen ways.

For example, let us reflect on pleasure and link the issue of pleasure with the three levels of experience introduced above. To begin on the mythological level, one sees that historically, the experience of pleasure has been an important part of human psychic experience, expressed through rituals. For example, humankind's first experience of pleasure, according to Greek mythology, was a joyous celebration. Pleasure had deep symbolic significance. In ancient times, Dionysus, the god of women, wine and joy, provided a collective way for women to experience ecstasy through a secret initiation rite acted out in the Villa of Mysteries in Pompeii.[10]

Given that mythology is somewhat lost in today's world, women do not have access to primitive experiences of ecstasy which can be found in myth and powerful, mythical images. In this light, the use of alcohol as an intoxicating substance may be for some women a replacement for a deep psychic need – the feeling of ecstasy. Abuse of alcohol may be one way in which a woman searches for a sense of exhilaration or enchantment but loses control of herself.

On the level of healing, pleasure can be linked with the development of autonomy, self-esteem and empowerment. But, real pleasure for women beyond the sexual tends to be invisible and denied in our society. In this context, women with drinking problems need to find pleasure in their healing. Here, pleasure becomes defined as moving towards something for oneself and it implies a certain amount of autonomy and self-worth. The words of Jean Kirkpatrick are instructive in this context: 'Emotional growth is happiness, spiritual growth is peace. Together these create a competent loving woman.'[11]

Susan Griffin contends that in our society women are seen as existing to provide pleasure to men and that women who survive are those who best succeed in pleasing men. In this light, drinking alcohol can be linked initially to a woman's way of giving pleasure to her body. For example, a woman who drinks a particular glass of champagne, wine or an exotic spirit can be viewed as sexy, attractive to men and a pleasurable sight for the male gaze. One only has to look at the shape of many drinking glasses, with their elegant curves and full, yet compact, shapes to sense the erotic, sexual connotations.[12] There are also mixed messages here. This is because a drunken woman is an unattractive woman and yet is seen as a potential sexual conquest – a slut.

In light of these comments, some women who confront problems with alcohol may be signalling a protest. They may be protesting the sexualised image of a woman with a glass in her hand. Feeling anxious about their role as pleasing men sexually or otherwise, they themselves may experience their overdrinking as unattractive. They may actually want to reject this sexualised image. Simply, their overdrinking may be a self-chosen way of saying 'no' to an oversexualized role. As we saw earlier, some women like the physical effects of alcohol on their bodies, as they develop their own 'boundaries'. The main point here is that in the initial stages, overdrinking may be a way of pleasing oneself and not others, including men. Unfortunately, this type of pleasure tends to backfire.

In the above discussion, the women and alcohol issue has been linked to myth, healing and the female body through the lens of pleasure. Other key areas of women's everyday lives besides pleasure may need to be unearthed and linked with these levels of experience in order to develop a full understanding of the women and alcohol issue. Nevertheless, this demonstrates how one can analyse other key areas of women's lives (such as work, caring, and so on) in relationship to these three important levels of experience.

To develop further the links between the woman and alcohol issue and these levels of experience, a brief discussion of the following related topics may be useful: Finding collective symbols through myths; Asserting oneself – a way of healing; and Social substance.

Finding collective symbols through myths

In looking closely at women's overdrinking, one may sense that somewhere within this experience there is social defiance. After all, women are not only involved in an activity which is defined as more male than female, but they are also putting their femininity at risk. On the one hand, by overdrinking, women are saying that they do not need to define themselves in relation to male values. On the other hand, they become deeply involved in supporting – whether directly or indirectly – men, masculinity and the male drinking culture. One woman describes this idea:

> Overdrinking behaviour is more for men. I always think that overdrinking women identify with men. For example, I imagine that they say to themselves, 'It is the aggressive man in me that is overdrinking. I am angry and I am going to drink. I have the image of the aggressive man in me.'

Related to these ideas, Jan Bauer uses myth to distinguish between what she calls an Athena and an Artemis conflict in women 'alcoholics'.[13] She contends that in private an overdrinking woman's collective role model is linked with Artemis, while in public it is linked with Athena. What does Bauer mean? Briefly, Artemis, the goddess of the woods, wild nature and women, is the model of a woman who does not define herself in terms of male values. On the other hand, as men's equal, Athena, the goddess of wisdom, is a male-supportive symbol; as Zeus' daughter she is most concerned with maintaining the Father Right, and protecting heroes. Women who consistently overdrink experience a conflict in themselves between rejecting male values and teaming up with men. For Bauer, women 'alcoholics' overcome this conflict, and in turn their overdrinking, by getting in touch with these opposite sides of themselves. As they learn to accept the creative sides of these goddesses as role models, they learn the full expression of their womanhood without alcohol.

This type of study may be helpful as well as fascinating for overdrinking women because they have few if any strong role models to emulate in society at large. The happy housewife, supermom and managerial woman have all been considered possible role models for contemporary women. But one wonders about the ultimate worth in aspiring to primarily male-defined role models. On the other hand, Bauer's mythological view of women and alcohol is more expansive. It allows women to see themselves in conflict, but in a conflict that can be resolved. Furthermore, in Bauer's approach, the experience of alcohol abuse becomes more closely linked to the creative sides of women's experience of themselves as women.

Asserting oneself – a way of healing

For women to gain power and strength is about demanding, organising and creating female space. This is not meant to suggest that women should separate totally from men, if they want female space – rather that women assert their right as autonomous persons to organise in women-only groups or women-only spaces separate from men. As we saw in Chapter Five, exploring this need for women-sensitive services in the alcohol field has been an important step towards the creation of women-sensitive ideas and practices. The atmosphere created by sharing experiences, problems and feelings is healing and transformative. In these spaces, women find the courage, hope and reassurance to understand and name their problems as their very own. For many overdrinking women, this gives them the strength to transform their lives.

The last thing any woman needs are supposedly healing experiences which make her feel worse. Bad experiences fuel a sense of self-hatred – not self-worth. As suggested in Chapter Four, if a woman seeks help and finds that she is treated in a less than respectful way, she will be damaged by that experience. Unfortunately, there are countless stories from women who have been ill-treated by treaters.[14] Treaters often attempt to transform their women patients into compliant female ex-alcoholics, with little regard for their needs.

These are the reasons why Jean Kirkpatrick founded Women for Sobriety as a programme to help a woman to 'affirm the value and worth of each woman', 'assert her belief in herself' and 'see herself in a positive and self-confident image'.[15]

In order to experience a sense of wholeness and healing, women are braving fragmented and isolated lives through alcohol. Throughout the discussions in this book the fact that women need to be deeply in touch with their creative powers has been underlined. With other women, they need to recognise their female integrity and transcend traditional and, at times, male-defined patterns of thinking, speaking and acting. Asserting oneself is all about focusing energy on oneself. In this healing process, stereotypical images that characterise women as diseased, neurotic, pathological, decadent or polluted are confronted and overturned. More important, women begin to search for alternative ways of preserving their female integrity, exercising their autonomy and expressing their rage.

Social substance

Discussions on the disease concept of alcohol revealed that this concept focused almost exclusively on men. In recent years, this disease concept was replaced by the 'alcohol dependence syndrome', the disease concept of alcohol in disguise. Usually, anything called a disease, including alcoholism (ie addiction dependency), is seen to be an impartial, organic thing living in the body of the diseased person. It is as if the diseased person lacks any social agency. Here, the concept of social substance may add a critical dimension to this traditional disease idea. It allows one to think abstractly as well as politically about alcoholism and, more important, it is sensitive to women.

Social substance is the significance that society gives to any individual's actions. It is all about how society evaluates one's social and moral agency. In this evaluation process, a system of ranking takes place based on gender as well as other forms of social inequality such as age, race, class, and so on. In the alcohol field, the concept of social substance permits one to consider how alcohol use and abuse affect an individual's social and moral agency. For example, people who drink portray moral as well immoral pictures. The moral picture is one of the moderate drinker, while the immoral picture is of the drunk. But regardless of the moral evaluation, these pictures are gendered. As we have seen, alcohol use tends to be a symbol of power for men and vulnerability for women – symbols that interact with social ideas on gendered bodies. Women's more than men's bodies as well as their moral and social agency appear to be more capable of corruption – more fragile. As a result, the social substance of women as a social group remains hidden, while their moral and social agency tends to be misunderstood, if not denied outright. This is not surprising given that historically the female body has been viewed as threatening to the moral and social stability of society.[16] Susan Griffin illustrates this idea and some of the deep misconceptions about women's social substance:

Her body is a vessel of death. Her beauty is a lure. . . . At the gate of her womb is a wound which bleeds freely. . . . She is mutilated. She is damaged. . . . She is a plague. A disease. . . . In her body is the seed of nothingness.[17]

Given the above discussion, it is perhaps easy to sense that resistance to a perspective sensitive to women will continue until outdated concepts are replaced by ones that reflect complex gendered processes. In seeking social substance, overdrinking women need to assert their moral and social agency. A first step would be to demand that they be evaluated on the same level as men, given that moral and social agency have had consistently different meanings for overdrinking men and women.

WOMEN AND ALCOHOL: EXPOSING NEW TENSIONS

Throughout this book, traditional views popular in the alcohol field have been challenged and replaced with a women-sensitive one. This is a minority view and reflects work by women and for women. But developing this view exposes unavoidable problems including the tension between an individualistic and a social approach to alcohol use, the power of the disease model and its effect on women, ideas on women and alcohol and women's everyday lives and, most important, the ideology of treaters defining how women should be treated and how this differs from the real needs of women.

Developing ideas and building theories in the alcohol field are mainly a male preserve. Nevertheless, male researchers and clinicians do use apparently 'gender sensitive' terms such as 'the family', 'gender', etc. In this way, many give lip service to women's needs, while ideas on the oppression of women, the need for women's autonomy and liberation, and social inequalities based on sex, race and class are mentioned in passing.

To develop a women-sensitive view requires hard work both on the level of theory and practice. This development must be framed with an awareness that there is a long history behind the development of insensitive ideas towards women 'alcoholics'. These ideas will not disappear overnight. Therefore, women themselves need to create an alternative perspective. Creating an alternative is a political choice. It involves recognising that insensitivity to women is widespread and supported by the general tendency to ignore social and political concerns regarding alcohol. The alcohol field is one in which many forms of social inequalities tend to be legitimised.

WOMEN AND ALCOHOL: WHAT CAN WE DEPEND ON?

The main aim of this book has been to introduce the reader to the key concepts and to develop a women-sensitive perspective in the field of alcohol. We have looked at the term 'substance use' and seen why this particular term is more relevant to women than the terms 'disease', 'addiction' and 'illness'. We saw that the use of this term is particularly relevant in the field of alcohol because women 'alcoholics' are more often than not viewed as being more socially and individually depraved, corrupt or wicked than men 'alcoholics'. This overriding view illustrates quite clearly a double standard in the field. Simply, there are different sets of drinking ethics, norms and standards of treatment for men and women. The words of the women quoted in this book have shown that this process of gendering why and how individuals drink has a damaging, if not debilitating, effect upon women. Drinking women are not only perceived as fallen and morally corrupt but also contained and captured within a powerful gendered trap. This subtle process, both invisible and insidious, must be challenged. If not, more women who suffer from overdrinking will continue to be hurt unnecessarily.

We also saw that alcohol is *the* social drug most widely used in society. This fact, linked with society's idea that a real 'alcoholic' is a man, tends to make women's problems secondary. A strong inclination to ignore overall social and political issues *vis-à-vis* women drinkers exists. As we have seen, those who hold the power to define women's problems in the alcohol field tend to be masculinist and apolitical, and thus they legitimate a whole series of social inequalities based on sex, race and class.

Hopefully, this book has shown our commonality as women as well as our differences. In this context, Adrienne Rich has said:

> Women both have and have not a common world. The mere sharing of oppression does not constitute a common world. Our thought and action, in so far as they have taken the form of difference, assertion, or rebellion, have repeatedly been obliterated, or subsumed under human history, which means the publicity of the public realm created and controlled by men.[18]

While women have often been erased within traditional studies in the alcohol field, we need powerful ideas which no longer allow erasure or subjugation in our public or private spaces. We already know that alcohol does not give us power. We give ourselves power. We take it. With this deeply cherished power, we come to understand our pain. We learn to overcome the invisible ban on women's enjoyment of life. As one insightful woman who has worked in this field said:

There are more rigid rules for women than men to use any desirable or addictive substance. In every country of the world, whether it is rich or poor, there are always places – like cafes, restaurants, or bars – where men gather. If the local men are not drinking alcohol, they are using something else. Maybe it is the one desirable substance in this country. But the men are taking it, drinking it, sniffing it or eating it. The women are not. The substance can be alcohol, cigarettes, cocaine – whatever. But women are not there and women are not encouraged to participate. This is because wherever one goes, women are not allowed to be seen to be enjoying themselves through substances or in any way. This is because we are born to be mothers – to be mothers for our children and to be mothers for the whole world. Women need to be taking care of other people. So how can any woman be just sitting there like a man and enjoying life. How can a woman enjoy life.

As we learn to overcome the invisible ban on women's enjoyment and continue building an alternative perspective on women and alcohol, we may want to convert the last sentence into a question, 'How can women enjoy life?' In asking this question, we want to learn what women can really depend on.

This book has attempted to demonstrate commonality as well as difference in a women-sensitive perspective on alcohol. Yes, the needs of women drinkers have been eradicated under the male-orientated public realm. Nevertheless, we shall slowly build ideas that refuse to allow women to be obliterated or subsumed in either the public or the private realm. Women, drinking in the privacy of the home or in public, may be perceived by men as endangering their femininity, partaking of a dangerous cocktail that threatens society's norms. But, perhaps, mixing women-sensitivity with alcohol is an even more dangerous social cocktail because it gives women the power both to understand and to act on that understanding.

Notes

1. Lesley Doyal, *What Makes Women Sick* (London: Macmillan, 1995), p 11.
2. This term comes from Rosi Briadoti's work 'Envy, or with Your Brains and My Looks', in A Jardine and R Smith, eds, *Men in Feminism* (London and New York: Methuen, 1987). The woman-in-me is that inner part of me as a woman which strives towards transcendence and spirituality – the things unseen.
3. For an interesting discussion of this tension, see J Kristeva, 'Oscillation between Power and Denial', in Elaine Marks and Isabelle de Courtivron. eds, *New French Feminists: An Anthology* (Brighton: Harvester Press, 1981).
4. See RW Connell, *Masculinities* (Berkeley, CA: University of California Press, 1995), p 71, where Connell begins to discuss gender as a structure of social practice.
5. See Susan Griffin, *Woman and Nature: The Roaring Inside Her* (London: The Women's Press, 1984), p 163.
6. These books have not been chosen arbitrarily. They are books that have informed my way of thinking about women and alcohol since the late 1980s.
7. Jan Bauer, *Alcoholism and Women: The Background and the Psychology* (Toronto: Inner City Books, 1982).
8. Jean Kirkpatrick, *Turnabout: New Help for the Woman Alcoholic* (Seattle: Madrona Publishers, 1986).
9. Susan Griffin, *Woman and Nature*.
10. See, for example, Linda Fierz-David, *Women's Dionysian Initiation: The Villa of Mysteries in Pompeii* (Dallas: Spring Publications, 1988), for a clear account of women's initiation ritual.
11. Jean Kirkpatrick, *Turnabout*, p 159.

12. Indeed, the way in which some brandy glasses are held may be suggestive of breast fondling.

13. Jan Bauer, *Alcoholism and Women*, pp 113–18.

14. See Peter Rutter, *Sex in the Forbidden Zone: When Men in Power – Therapists, Doctors, Clergy, Teachers, and Others – Betray Women's Trust* (London: Unwin Paperbacks, 1990), for accounts of abuse (sexual and otherwise) experienced by women in a variety of treatment settings.

15. Jean Kirkpatrick, *Turnabout*, p 162.

16. For an interesting and gender-sensitive discussion of this idea, see Bryan S Turner, *Medical Power and Social Knowledge* (London: Sage, 1987), pp 85–87.

17. Susan Griffin, *Woman and Nature*, pp 83–84.

18. Adrienne Rich, 'Foreword: Conditions for Work: The Common World of Women', in Sara Ruddick and Pamela Daniels, eds, *Working It Out* (New York: Pantheon Books, 1977), pp xiii-xxiv.

BIBLIOGRAPHY

Alcohol Concern, *Women and Drinking*, Alcohol Concern, London, 1988.

Alcoholics Anonymous, *The AA Way of Life: A Reader by Bill*, AA Publishing Company, London, 1967.

— *The Story of How Many Thousands of Men and Women Have Recovered from Alcoholism*, Hazell, Watson and Viney, Aylesbury, UK, 1963.

— *Twelve Steps and Twelve Traditions*, Hazell, Watson and Viney, Aylesbury, UK, 1974.

Atwood, JD and Randall, T, 'Domestic Violence: The Role of Alcohol', *Journal of the American Medical Association* 255 (4)1991, pp 460–61.

Bartsky, Sandra Lee, *Feminism and Domination*, Routledge, New York and London, 1990.

Bauer, Jan, *Alcoholism and Women: The Background and the Psychology*, Inner City Books, Toronto, 1982.

Beckman, Linda J, 'Women Alcoholics: A Review of Social and Psychological Studies', *Journal of the Studies of Alcohol* 36, 1975, pp 797–824.

Bepko, Claudia (ed), *Feminism and Addiction*, The Haworth Press, New York, London and Sydney, 1991.

Berenson, David, 'Powerlessness-liberating or Enslaving? Responding to the Feminist Critique of the Twelve Steps', in Bepko, Claudia (ed), *Feminism and Addiction*, The Haworth Press, New York, London and Sydney, 1991.

Björling, Bam, 'Making Women Visible', in Haavio-Mannila, Elina (ed), *Women, Alcohol and Drugs in the Nordic Countries*, Nordic Council for Alcohol and Drug Research, Helsinki, 1989.

Bolen, Jean Shinoda, *Goddesses in Everywoman: A New Psychology of Women*, Harper and Row Publishers, New York, 1985.

Boothroyd, Wilfred E, 'Nature and Development of Alcoholism in Women' in Kalant, Orian Josseau (ed), *Research Advance in Alcohol and Drug Problems, Volume 5, Alcohol and Drug Problems in Women*, Plenum Press, London and New York, 1980.

Bovey, Shelly, *Being Fat Is not a Sin*, Pandora, London, 1989.

Briadoti, Rosi, 'Envy, or with Your Brains and My Looks', in Jardine, A, and Smith, R (eds), *Men in Feminism*, Methuen, London and New York, 1987.

Camberwell Council on Alcoholism, *Women and Alcohol*, Tavistock, London and New York, 1980.

Chernin, Kim, *The Hungry Self: Women, Eating and Identity*, Virago, London, 1985.

Connell, RW, *Masculinities*, University of California Press, Berkeley, CA, 1995.

Day, Nancy L, 'The Effects of Prenatal Exposure to Alcohol', in *Alcohol World and Health Research* 10,1992, p 3.

Douglas, Mary (ed), *Constructive Drinking: Perspectives on Drink from Anthropology*, Cambridge University Press, Cambridge, 1987.

Douglas, Mary, *Purity and Danger: An Analysis of Pollution and Taboo*, Routledge and Kegan Paul, London and Henley, 1966.

Dowrick, Stephanie, *The Intimacy and Solitude Self-Therapy Book*, The Women's Press, London, 1993.

Doyal, Lesley, *What Makes Women Sick*, Macmillan, London, 1995.

Duckert, Fanny, 'The Treatment of Female Problem Drinkers' in Haavio-Mannila, Elina (ed), *Women, Alcohol and Drugs in the Nordic Countries*, Nordic Council for Alcohol and Drug Research, Helsinki, 1989.

Ernst, Sheila, and Goodison, Lucy, *In Our Own Hands: A Book of Self-Help Therapy*, The Women's Press, London, 1981.

Ettorre, Dr EM, *A Survey of Facilities for Women Using Drugs (Including Alcohol)*, DAWN, London, 1985.

Ettorre, Elizabeth, 'Substance Use and Women's Health', in Wilkinson, Sue, and Kitzinger, Celia (eds), *Women and Health: Feminist Perspectives*, Taylor and Francis, London, 1994.

— *Women and Substance Use*, Macmillan, London, and Rutgers University Press, New Brunswick, NJ, 1992.

Ettorre, EM, 'Self-Help Groups as an Alternative to Benzodiazepine Use', in Gabe, Jonathan, and Williams, Paul (eds), *Tranquillisers: Social,*

Psychological and Clinical Perspectives, Tavistock, London, 1986.

Faderman, Lillian, *Odd Girls and Twilight Lovers: A History of Lesbian Life in Twentieth-Century America*, Viking Penguin, New York, 1991.

Fierz-David, Linda, *Women's Dionysian Initiation: The Villa of Mysteries in Pompeii*, Spring Publications, Dallas, 1988.

Fillmore, KM, 'When Angels Fall: Women's Drinking as Cultural Preoccupation and as Reality', in Wilsnack, SC, and Beckman, L (eds), *Alcohol Problems in Women: Antecedents and Consequences*, Guilford Press, New York, 1984.

Forth-Finegan, JL, 'Sugar and Spice and Everything Nice: Gender Socialization and Women's Addiction – A Literature Review' in Bepko, Claudia (ed), *Feminism and Addiction*, The Haworth Press, New York, London and Sydney, 1991.

Gefou-Madianou, Dimitra (ed), *Alcohol, Gender and Culture*, Routledge, New York and London, 1992.

Gefou-Madianou, Dimitra, 'Alcohol Commensality, Identity Transformations and Transcendence' in Gefou-Madianou, Dimitra (ed), *Alcohol, Gender and Culture*, Routledge, New York and London, 1992.

Glatt, Max, *Alcoholism*, Hodder and Stoughton, Sevenoaks, UK, 1982.

Graham, Hilary, 'The Concept of Caring in Feminist Research: The Case of Domestic Service', *Sociology* 25 (1), pp 61-78.

Griffin, Susan, *Woman and Nature: The Roaring Inside Her*, The Women's Press, London, 1984.

Hafner, Sarah, *Nice Girls Don't Drink: Stories of Recovery*, Bergin and Garvey, New York, 1992.

Hall, Nor, *The Moon and the Virgin*, The Women's Press, London, 1980.

Harper, CG, Smith, NA and Krill, JJ, 'The Effects of Alcohol on the Human Brain: A Neuropathological Study', *Alcohol* 25,1990, pp 445–48.

Harwin, J, and Otto, S, 'Women, Alcohol and the Screen', in Cook, J, and Lewington, M (eds), *Images of Alcoholism*, British Film Institute and Alcohol Education Centre, London, 1979.

Hirschmann, JR, and Munter, CH, *Overcoming Overeating*, Fawcett Columbine, New York, 1988.

Jellinek, EM, *The Disease Concept of Alcoholism*, College and University Press in association with Hillhouse Press, New Haven, CT, 1960.

Jones, KL, and Smith, DW, 'Recognition of the Foetal Alcohol Syndrome in Early Infancy', *Lancet* 2, 1973, pp 999–1001.

Kent, Rosemary, *Say When!: Everything a Woman Needs to Know about Alcohol and Drinking Problems*, Sheldon Press, London, 1990.

Kirkpatrick, Jean, *Turnabout: New Help for the Woman Alcoholic*, Madrona Publishers, Seattle, 1986.

Krestan, J, and Bepko, Claudia, 'Codependency: The Social Reconstruction of Female Experience' in Bepko, Claudia (ed), *Femininism and Addiction*, The Haworth Press, New York, London and Sydney, 1991.

Kristeva, J, 'Oscillation between Power and Denial', in Marks, Elaine, and de Courtivron, Isabelle (eds), *New French Feminists: An Anthology*, Harvester Press, Brighton, 1981.

Lauy, G, 'Nutmeg Intoxication in Pregnancy: A Case Report', *Journal of Reproductive Medicine* 32,1,1987, pp 63–64.

Mason, M, 'Women and Shame: Kin and Culture' in Bepko, Claudia (ed), *Feminism and Addiction*, The Haworth Press, New York, London and Sydney, 1991.

Mason, Marilyn, 'Women and Shame: Kin and Culture' in Bepko, Claudia (ed), *Feminism and Addiction*, The Haworth Press, New York, London and Sydney, 1991.

McConville, Brigid, *Women Under the Influence: Alcohol and its Impact*, Shocken Books, New York, 1983.

McDonald, Maryon (ed), *Gender, Drink and Drugs*, Berg Publishers, Oxford, 1994.

McIntyre, Jeffrey, 'Reflections on Male Codependency' in Bepko, Claudia (ed), *Feminism and Addiction*, The Haworth Press, New York, London and Sydney, 1991.

Miller, Dusty, 'Are We Keeping up with Oprah?: A Treatment and Training Model for Addictions and Interpersonal Violence' in Bepko, Claudia (ed), *Feminism and Addiction*, The Haworth Press, New York, London and Sydney, 1991.

Murphy, S, and Rosenbaum, M, 'Editors' Introduction', *Journal of Psychoactive Drugs* 19, 2, 1987, pp 125–28.

Norton, R, Dwyer, T and Macmahon, S, 'Alcohol Consumption and the Risk of Alcohol Related Cirrhosis in Women', *British Medical Journal* 295, 1987, pp 80–82.

Oakley, Ann, *The Captured Womb: A History of the Medical Care of Pregnant Women*, Basil Blackwell, Oxford, 1984.

Orbach, Susie, *Fat Is a Feminist Issue*, Hamlyn Publications, London, 1978.

— *Hunger Strike*, Faber and Faber, London, 1986.

Otto, Shirley, 'Single Homeless Women and Alcohol' in Camberwell Council on Alcoholism, *Women and Alcohol*, Tavistock, London and

New York, 1980.

Pancoast, DL, Parker, P, and Froland, C (eds), *Rediscovering Self-Help: Its Role in Social Care*, Sage Publications, Beverly Hills, CA, 1983.

Pasick, Patricia, and White, Christine, 'Challenging General Patton: A Feminist Stance in Substance Abuse Treatment and Training' in Bepko, Claudia (ed), *Feminism and Addiction*, The Haworth Press, New York, London and Sydney, 1991.

Plant, Moira, *Women, Drinking and Pregnancy*, Tavistock, London, 1985.

Raymond, Janice, *A Passion for Friends: Toward a Philosophy of Female Affection*, The Women's Press, 1986.

Rich, Adrienne, 'Foreword: Conditions for Work: The Common World of Women' in Ruddick, Sara, and Daniels, Pamela (eds), *Working It Out*, Pantheon Books, New York, 1977.

Robertson, I, and Heather, N, *Let's Drink to Your Health*, British Psychological Society, Leicester, 1986.

Room, Robin, 'Alcohol as an Instrument of Intimate Domination', paper presented to the Society for the Study of Social Problems Annual Meeting, New York, August 1980.

Rose, Hilary, *Love, Power and Knowledge*, Polity Press, Cambridge, 1994.

Rosett, HL, 'The Effects of Alcohol on the Fetus and Offspring', in Kalant, OJ (ed), *Alcohol and Drug Problems in Women*, Plenum Press, New York and London, 1980.

Royal College of Psychiatrists, *Alcohol and Alcoholism: Report of a Special Commission*, Tavistock, London, 1979.

Rutter, Peter, *Sex in the Forbidden Zone: When Men in Power – Therapists, Doctors, Clergy, Teachers, and Others – Betray Women's Trust*, Unwin Paperbacks, London, 1990.

Sandmair, M, *The Invisible Alcoholics: Women and Alcohol Abuse in America*, McGraw Hill, New York, 1980.

Sarachild, Kathie, 'Consciousness Raising: A Radical Weapon' in Sarachild, Kathie (ed) *Feminist Revolution*, Radstockings, New York, 1975.

Sargent, Margaret, *Women, Drugs and Policy in Sydney, London and Amsterdam*, Avebury Press, Aldershot, UK, 1992.

Schaef, AW, *Co-dependence: Misunderstood – Mistreated*, Winston Press, Minneapolis, 1986.

Schoenfield, Lisa, and Wieser, Barb (eds), *Shadow on a Tightrope: Writings by Women on Fat Oppression*, Aunt Lute Book Company, Iowa City, IA, 1983.

Sloven, Jane, 'Codependent or Empathically Responsive?: Two Views of

Betty', in Bepko, Claudia (ed), *Feminism and Addiction*, The Haworth Press, New York, London and Sydney, 1991.

Smith, Dorothy, *Texts, Facts and Femininity: Exploring the Relations of Ruling*, Routledge, London, 1990.

Sontage, LN, and Wallace, RF, 'The Effect of Smoking During Pregnancy on the Fetal Heart Rate', *American Journal of Obstetrics and Gynecology* 29, 1935, pp 77–83.

Thom, Betsy, 'Women and Alcohol: The Emergence of a Risk Group', in McDonald, Maryon (ed), *Gender, Drink and Drugs*, Berg, Oxford, 1994.

Turner, Bryan S, *Medical Power and Social Knowledge*, Sage, London, 1987.

van Wormer, Katherine, *Alcoholism Treatment: A Social Work Perspective*, Nelson Hall Publishers, Chicago, 1995.

Walker, G, Eric, Kathleen, Pivnick, A, and Drucker, E, 'A Descriptive Outline of a Program for Cocaine-using Mothers and their Babies' in Bepko, Claudia (ed), *Feminism and Addiction*, The Haworth Press, New York, London and Sydney, 1991.

Waterson, Jan, and Ettorre, Betsy, 'Providing Services for Women with Difficulties with Alcohol and Other Drugs: The Current UK Situation as Seen by Women Practitioners, Researchers and Policy Makers in the Field', *Drug and Alcohol Dependence* 24, 1989, pp 119–25.

Woodman, Marion, *Addiction to Perfection: The Still Unravished Bride*, Inner City Books, Toronto, 1982.

INDEX

numbers in brackets refer to *notes*

The Women's Press is Britain's leading women's publishing house. Established in 1978, we publish high-quality fiction and non-fiction from outstanding women writers worldwide. Our exciting and diverse list includes literary fiction, detective novels, biography and autobiography, health, women's studies, handbooks, literary criticism, psychology and self help, the arts, our popular Livewire Books series for young women and the bestselling annual *Women Artists Diary* featuring beautiful colour and black-and-white illustrations from the best in contemporary women's art.

If you would like more information about our books or about our mail order book club, please send an A5 sae for our latest catalogue and complete list to:

The Sales Department
The Women's Press Ltd
34 Great Sutton Street
London EC1V 0DX
Tel: 0171 251 3007
Fax: 0171 608 1938